THE SCIENCE OF PULSE EXAMINATION IN AYURVEDA

Indian Medical Science Series No. 57

THE SCIENCE OF PULSE EXAMINATION IN AYURVEDA

Vaidya Govind Prasad Upadhyay
M.D. (Ay.)

Published by:
Sri Satguru Publications
Indological and Oriental Publishers
A Division of
Indian Books Centre
40/5, Shakti Nagar,
Delhi-110007
(INDIA)

First Edition : Delhi, 1997

ISBN 81-7030-539-X

Printed in India.

Published by Sunil Gupta, for Sri Satguru Publications, a division of Indian Books Centre, 40/5, Shakti Nagar, Delhi-110007, India, and printed at D.K. Fine Art Press, Delhi-110052.

Preface

After the publication of my 'Siddhida' Hindi Commentary, on Ravana's 'Nadi Pariksha' many scholars advised me to write an independent text on pulse examination. While translating or writing a commentary, a writer is bound within certain limitations. One has to abide by the chronological order present in the original text. The books which are available today on pulse examination show a lack of uniformity and order. Hence keeping the above factors in mind, the book 'Science of Pulse Examination' is dedicated to the world of Ayurveda.

'Nadi Pariksha' or pulse examination has been synonymous with diagnosis in Ayurveda. Whenever a patient goes for consultation to a physician, he says, `I am going to the physician for pulse examination.' Surely this science might have developed and enjoyed acceptance in masses. History bears testimony to it in ample measure.

The fact cannot be denied that a planned attempt was made to destroy the Ayurvedic science along with other Indian traditional arts during alien rules. In comparison to the popularity of pulse examination, utility in clinical practice, prevalent, available literature is rare. The increasing tendency in modern diagnostic techniques, the uncertainity and the high cost involved in the modern science again directed the attention of medical world towards the science of pulse examination'. Responding to the need of western medical world, the book is being presented in English. 'Science of Pulse Examination.' Emphasis is given to practical approach based on experiences with comprehensive compilation of ancient references and scientific presentation. This book is an humble attempt in this direction

There are different opinions in Ayurveda itself regarding `Pulse Examination'. According to some scholars pulse examination is very authentic and useful in practice but some others have an opinion that there is exaggeration in this regard, and it has limited diagnostic scope. Rational analysis brings us to the following conclusion:

1. This science has survived through ages even in adverse circumstances which proves the utility of this science.

2. Even if we leave apart the historical evidence and the epigrams, many persons have themselves seen the senior Ayurvedic physicians diagnosing accurately with pulse examination alone. Not only this, with the help of pulse examination they have been able to state the outstanding facts of patients' personal history aetiopathogenesis, psychological condition, prognosis of the disease, etc. This underlines inadequancy in human competence rather than science itself.

3. Pulse examination is necessary for the poor, dumb, deaf, lunatic, and imbecile patients, for immediate diagnosis, in developing regions.

4. It is imperative to accept the rationality of science of pulse examination not only for the welfare of the society but medical science as well.

5. There is a need to develop the science of pulse examination with new interpretations.

It is my fortune that Shri Vd. Tarashanker Mishra author of the famous book 'Nadi Darshan' and Shri Vd. Vishwanath Dwivedi, author of 'Abhinav Nadi Tantra' have been my gurus. It is my privilege that I had the opportunity to learn this science from Shri vd. Kashinath Shastri and Shri Vd. Yadunandan Upadhyay a direct disciple of Vd. Satyanarayan Shastri. The blessings of these Acharyas are real treasure in my life. I am deeply indebted to them. I am indeed grateful to Prof. R.H. Singh (B.H.U.) for his Foreword.

In my maiden attempt to author a volume on Pulse Examination in English deficencies are unavoidable. I look forward to criticisms and suggestins from readers for corrective measures in next edition, which would be gratefully acknowledged.

I am thankful to Miss Vandana Savant and Miss Manju Mishra for their kind cooperation in preparation of this manuscript.

G.P. Upadhyay
Reader & Head of the Deptt.
Deptt. of Roga Nidan-VikritiVigyan
Shri Ayurved Mahvidyalya
Nagpur– (Maharashtra)

Contents

FOREWORD

Ayurveda is one of the most ancient medical sciences of the world. Certain authorities consider Ayurveda as the Upaveda of Atharva Veda and as such its antiquity goes back to Vedas, the earliest recorded wisdom on the earth. The good old knowledge of Ayurveda is survived to the modern age in the form of two sets of authentic classic texts of three books each, popularly called the *Vrhattrayee* and *Laghuttrayee*. These texts, besides the preclinical basic aspects of Ayurveda, describe in detail the theory and practice of Eight clinical specialities namely *Kayachikitsa* (Internal Medicine), *Shalya Tantra* (Surgery), *Shalakya Tantra* (Opthalmology and ENT), *Kaumarbhrita* (Maternity and child health), *Rasayana* (Geriatrics), *Vajikarana* (Sexology), *Agada Tantra* (Toxicology) and *Bhutavidya* (Psychiatry). These Eight desciplines represent Clinical Ayurveda which is well supported by preclinical Ayurvedic sciences like fundamental principles, Ayurvedic pharmacology and pharmaceutics. The Ayurvedic texts describe in detail the diagnostic methodology to be used by the above a eight kinds of physicians and surgeons in patient care.

Ayurvedic treatment fundamentally intends to disintegrate the disease process by *Samprapti Vighatana* leading to restoration of Normalcy i.e. *Prakriti Sthapana*. Ayurvedic diagnostics is not limited only to identifying the specific disease by a `Name'. It advocates to endeavour for a detailed information about the disease phenomenon and its constituent morbid factors so that adequate measures may be instituted for total cure. The following statement of Charaka is of special significance in this context which emphasises that neither it is possible nor necessary to give `Name' to every disease state. Each disease state needs separate descriptive identification in each individual.

विकारनामाकुशलो न जिह्रीयात्कदाचन।
न हि सर्वविकाराणां नामतोऽस्ति ध्रुवा स्थितिः।।   चरक सूत्र 18: 44

In view of the above approach Ayurveda advocates for a very detailed clinical examination of a patient. It does not believe in any short cut in diagnosis. The classical Ayurveda also does not suggest to make full and finial diagnosis only by *Nadi Pariksha,* which some times is claimed by certain contemporary Vaidyas. *Mystics,* miracles and short cuts are against the spirit of broad based diagnostic approach of Ayurveda. Besides, Ayurveda also pleads for a very superior quality of rapport between the patient and the doctor as is evident from the following verse quoted from Charaka.

ज्ञान बुद्धि प्रदीपेन यो नाविशति तत्वविद् ।
आतुरस्यान्तरात्मानं न स रोगाश चिकित्सति ।। चरक वि॰ 4.

Another important originality and superiority of Ayurvedic diagnostics is its two fold approach identifying *Roga* and *Rogi* separately where emphasis is given in the study of the basic nature of the patient and his remainder health for which detailed *Dasavidha Pariksha is described by Charaka*. The disease state is examined in Ayurvedic practice by *Prashna Pariksha* or interrogation and *Panchendriya Pariksha* or physical Examination. In the ethos of such a broad based approach of Ayurveda it is intriguing how and from where the claims of short cut diagnosis by Pulse reading alone crept in.

It is interesting to note that *Nadi Pariksha* has not been even mentioned in Ayurvedic Classics. The first glimpse of this art is seen in the texts of late medieval period like *Yoga Ratnakara* and *Sharangdhara Samhita* when *Nadi Pariksha* entered into the main stream of Clinical Medicine by way of *Astavidha Pariksha* where *Nadi* was mentioned on priority one among the eight points to be examined.

रोगाक्रान्त शरीरस्य स्थानान्यष्टौ परीक्षयेत् ।
नाड़ी मूत्रं मलं जिह्वां शब्दं स्पर्श दृगाकृति ।। यो॰ र॰

In this context the Acharyas have described in certain details the concepts and practical details of pulse reading with *Tridoshik* correlates characteristically comparing *Vatika, Paittika* and *Kaphaja Nadis* with *Sarpa Gati* (crawling of a snake), *Manduka Gati* (jumping of a frog) and *Hansa Gati* (full walk of a swan) respectively. *Nadi Pariksha* is more an Art and perceptual concentration than simple clinical technique.

The author of the present monograph Dr. Govind Prasad Upadhyaya has done full justice to this handy write-up on the important topic of *Nadi Parkisha*. He has ably incorporated the available textual references from all sources with suitable codification and interpretation in the light of his clinical experience. Dr. Upadhyaya is known to me for about two decades. He started his career as a postgraduate student under me in late seventies at Banaras Hindu University and rapidly grew in his academic and professional stature and presently happens to be one of the most brilliant Ayurvedists in the country. I congratulate him for producing this interesting monograph and wish all the best in his career.

(Prof. R.H. Singh)
Professor & Head
Department of Kayachikitsa
Institute of Medical Sciences
Banaras Hindu University
VARANASI-221005
INDIA

1

Science of Pulse Examination

In each and every medical science of the world there is a method to examine the pulse of a patient. But the detailed study of pulse examination is found only in Ayurveda. No other science has dealt it with so much profoundness. In Ayurveda, Pulse examination has become a synonym for 'diagnosis'. When a patient comes to a physician then without much delay he stretches his hand so that the physician examines his pulse and diagnoses his disease. There have been some physicians who used to examine the pulse of the patient and were able to tell the etiology, symptoms and prognosis of disease.

From the historical point of view the knowledge of pulse examination is found during the medieval period (13 to 16th century), In Vedic and Sanhita period (2000 B.C. to 8th century) the word 'Nadi' has been mentioned but scientific description of pulse examination is not available.

Normally the word 'Nadi' and 'Nadi Sansthan' stand for nerves and nervous system respectively, but in Ayurveda 'Nadi Tu Dhamani Sira' which implies that the word 'Nadi' stands for blood vessels as well. The word 'Nadi' has also been used in the context of network of blood capillaries. In this way the word 'Nadi' stands for different meanings but the term 'Pulse examination' means a careful planned test carried out by the physician for diagnosis of disease.

Some scholars are of the view that the science of Pulse Examination has been borrowed from the Greek Medical Science. This is because the science of Pulse Examination has been found in detail in the literatures found in 'Sangraha' period. The reason for this is probably that it was the Mughal rule when the texts on Ayurveda were translated in Arabic & Persian languages. It is quite possible that the Greek literature was also translated in Sanskrit and Hindi. Thus, there was an exchange of knowledge, ideas etc. But the method of pulse examination found in Greek texts and Hindu texts are not identical. In fact there is a conceptual difference. From historical point of view, Ayurvedic books which deal with the science of pulse examination were written much before the Mughal era. Thus it is very clear that the method of pulse examination found in Ayurveda is a developed science rooted in Ayurveda and not derived or borrowed.

The contribution of 'Bhartiya Yoga' and 'Tantra Shastra' has helped in the development of the science of pulse examination. The word 'Nadi' has been technically used in books as 'Ida, Pingla' etc. The origin of terms such a Nabhi Chakra, Hrithkamal, Koorma, Kundalini, Chitta-Bhoomi etc. found in Ayurveda have their origin in the 'Tantra & Yoga' scriptures.

The methodology of examination of a patient is an independent science. The science of examining a patient by touch (sparshan) is an integral part of clinical examination which includes examination of the organs by palpation & percussion. The science of pulse examination becomes a part of 'Sparshan Pariksha'. The acceptance of pulse examination by the physician led to the gradual development of this science. Above all the contribution of 'Yogashastra', 'Tantra vigyan' in ample measure paved way for its comprehensive development. Acharyas like Ravana and Kanad who wrote independent texts in addition to Yog Ratnakar and Sharangdhar who devoted independent chapters, successfully contributed to the total acceptance of this science. Pulse examination is a practical science which became popular and controversial depending upon the social and educational status of Ayurveda. The decline of the Guru-Shishya tradition and increasing haste in life have made this science unacceptable. Prevailing increase in laboratory investigation has led to decline of other traditional methods along with the science of Pulse examination. But due to heavy expenses in laboratory investigation and the development of doubts in certain areas have again attracted the attention of practitioner towards the science of pulse examination. The science of pulse examination is a boon for the poor in developing countries.

Important and acceptance of Pulse Examination:-

Pulse examination is basis of diagnosis in Ayurveda. Pulse examination is supposed to be an alternative approach to diagnose the diseases. Disease dwells in unhealthy body. Certain noticeable changes develope in the patients body which help the physician in the diagnosis. Physicians have described 8-parts of body where the physical manifestations can be noticed.

The following eight parts of a patient should be examined–pulse, urine, faeces, tongue, voice, touch, eyes and physique (shape). A controversy is seen in this, but in eight fold examination physicians have invariably accepted examination of the pulse as the first step. Other examinations reveal the disorder at a particular region in a limited way but the examination of pulse is of fundmental importance in all disorders. Following reasons underline the importance of pulse examination:

1. This examination is done externally without disturbing any internal system.
2. Pulse examination does not require any physical, chemical or electrical instrument. Darkness, light, heat, cold do not affect it in any way.
3. The physician himself examines the pulse and correlates with the symptoms and takes the decisions accordingly.
4. Infant, females, imbecile, dumb, paralysed, comatose, infirm, lunatic etc. who are unable to communicate their diseases to the physician can take the advantage of pulse examination.
5. It is not expensive.
6. It does not require much time for diagnosis.
7. Now a days biochemical tests are expensive and time consuming. Physical pain has to be born by the patients. It is not easily available. Reports are produced by other persons whereas pulse examination saves time and money and without physical pain to the patient. The physician examines the pulse himself.
8. Pulse examination can be done during wars, accidents, floods, heavy rains and at places where equipments are not availabl
9. It is equally useful for undeveloped and developed countries.
10. The education and training of pulse examination is not only simple and easy to practice but economical too. Trainees can become skilled by practice while other methods require expensive training.

11. The decrease, increase and equilibrium of the Doshas can be known.
12. Normally for most of the diseases this practice is convenient and important.
13. Apart from the diagnosis the physician comes to know the characteristics, the nature and the extent of the disease with all its pathological implications.
14. The knowledge of combination (anubandhta) of 'Doshas' in different diseases is also obtained.
15. Apart from the causes of disease Pulse Examination also reveals the diet of the person.
16. It helps in differential diagnosis.
17. Pulse examination also gives an idea of the mental state of the patient i.e. tension, sorrow, anger, lust, greed, depression etc.
18. It also helps in detecting symptoms of progress and prognosis.
19. A physician is able to decide whether the disease is curable or incurable.
20. It tells us about "Sama" and "Nirama".
21. A physician can predict the gender of the foetus.
22. Response to treatment can be assessed by pulse examination.

2

Methodology of Pulse Examination

Pulse examination is a technical procedure which has a specific methodology. The method of pulse examination according to the texts is divided in three categories:

1. Relating to the physician.
2. Relating to the patients.
3. Relating to the method of examination.

Full knowledge, and a correct decision can be taken only by adherance to above aspects. Some rules are very important which cannot be neglected during pulse examinations while others can be adopted according to the circumstances. For example:- If a patient has been affected by heat or cold a few moments back then the results which are affected by this fact can be neglected.

Relating to the Physician:

1. A physician should sit with a sound stable mind and examine the pulse with concentration.
2. A physician must be healthy in body and mind. If he himself is ailing or unhealthy then he will not be able to examine the patient. Anger, greed, lust, depression etc. will hinde the physician in the diagnosis of patients.
3. For examining the pulse, a physician should sit comfortably facing towards north or east.
4. A physician should sit with a cheerful mood for examining the pulse.
5. A physician should not consume intoxicants such as alcohol during pulse examination.
6. The excretory system of the physician should be sound otherwise the physician will not be able to concentrate.
7. Physicians who are greedy and cherish various desires cannot examine the pulse successfully and so they should refrain themselves from the various cravings of the world.

8. A physician should use the three fingers of his right hand to examine the pulse.
9. If his hands are cold then heat should be generated by mutual friction of hands.
10. Eagerness is not required during pulse examination. The pulse should be examined for two minutes at least.

Relating to the Patient:

1. The patient should be free from the excretory products of the body.
2. The patient should sit comfortably with folded hands or must lie comfortably on the bed and then examined.
3. The pulse of a patient who is sleeping must not be examined.
4. The pulse of a patient who is hungry or thirsty must not be examined.
5. The pulse of a patient should not be examined just after the meals.
6. The pulse of a patient who has come directly from the sun must not be examined immediately.
7. The pulse of a patient who has taken his bath or had excercises must not be examined immediately.
8. The patient should not have indulged in intercourse.
9. The patient should not be on a fast (hungry).
10. The patient should not have consumed intoxicant.
11. Pulse should not examined during 'Bhootavishta' and epileptical attacks (influenced with external factors).
12. If a patient has lust, sorrow, greed, fear, depression or anxiety in his mind, then the pulse should not be examined. He must be calmed and then examined.
13. Patient affected by extreme cold, extreme heat, stimulants must not be subjected to pulse examination.
14. The pulse should not be examined with patient in standing position.

Due to above reasons, the pulse rate cannot be determined. "Samyag nadi na budhyate" imply that the diet, etiology, psychological conditions affect the pulse rate and so the disease and its vitiation cannot be known. If the patient has not defecated or urinated, it results in increase in activity of "Vata" Dosha which in turn affects the pulse rate. So the patient must become free from excretion during pulse examination.

Relating to Examination:

1. It is an ancient tradition to examine the pulse in the morning with empty stomach.
2. The patient should sit or lie down comfortably and then be examined.
3. A patient's hand should be relaxed and slightly flexed.
4. If a patient is sitting then the physician must give the support of his left hand below the elbow joint in order to make the hand relaxed and feel the pulse with ease.
5. The fingers of the patients should be quarterflexed just like a banana.
6. The stress or pressure on the radial artery must be removed. Under of stress or pressure the pulse is not feel normally.
7. The pulse of left hand in case of woman while the pulse of right hand of men should be examined. The best thing to do is that the pulse of both the hands must be examined. It may happen that the pulse rate of both hands may be different, therefore the pulse of right hand of men be checked first and then that of the left hand must be examined and vice versa for women.
8. A physician must use his index finger, middle finger and ring finger for pulse examination. He should put his fingers one by one with a slight pressure to find out the pulse rate.
9. The pulsation should be checked for one minute and not for fifteen seconds and then multiplied by four.
10. If a patient has taken tea, coffee, alcohol, cigarette, drugs etc. then there is an increase in pulse rate. On the other hand consumption of cold drinks, curd etc. leads to decrease in pulse rate.

11. An excited, tense or frightened patient need be calmed to normal mental composure with assurance, and then examined.
12. If the pulse at the wrist carries a doubt or is unclear then the pulses at various other places need be checked and then correlated.
13. Fingers kept on the pulse must be lifted and then again be kept with a slight pressure. This must be done at least three times and then the fractions of Doshic abnormality be assessed.
14. The hands of the patient who is lying must be a little curved and kept laterally facing towards the body.
15. If there is a doubt in the pulse rate then the physician must use a stethoscope and check the heart beat and the pulse rate.
16. If there is a doubt about the force then the pulse of both the hands must be examined simultaneously with both the hands of physician.

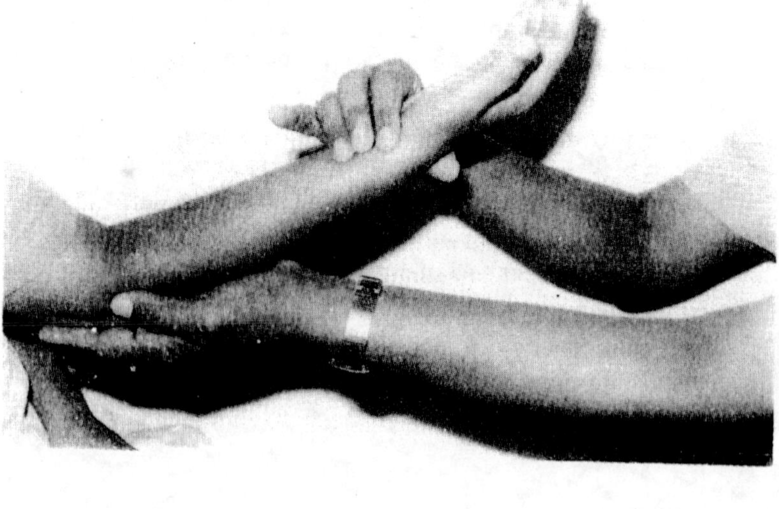

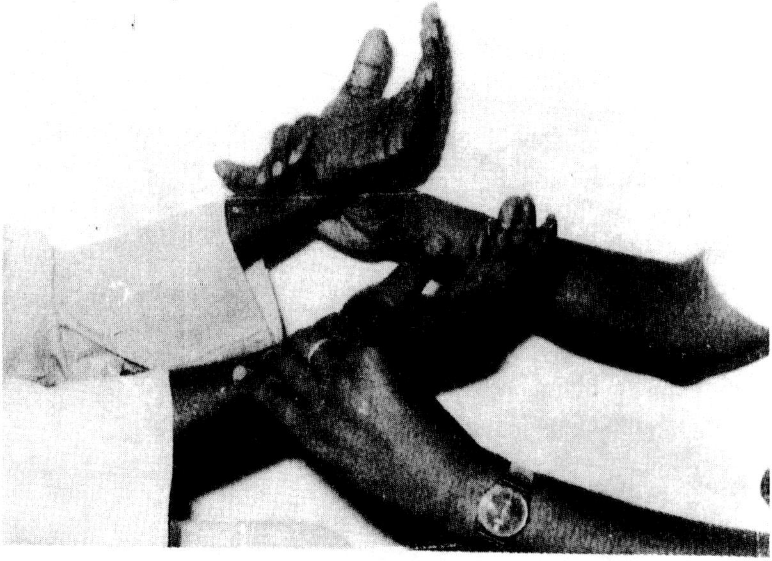

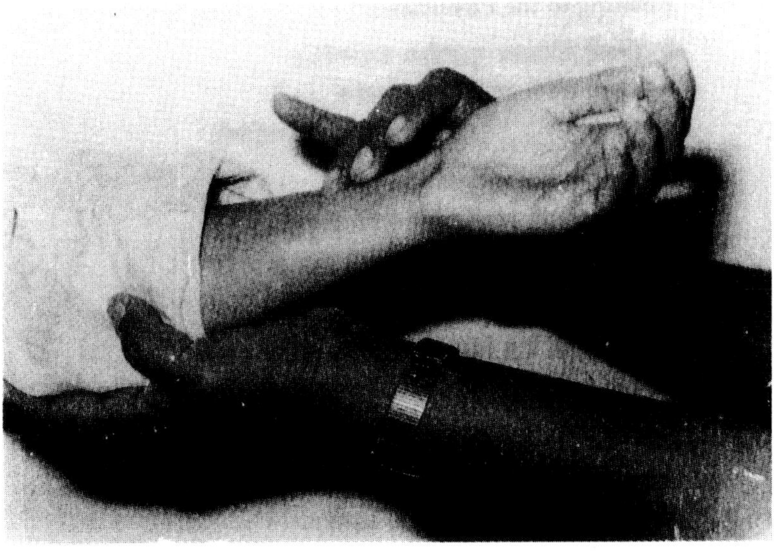

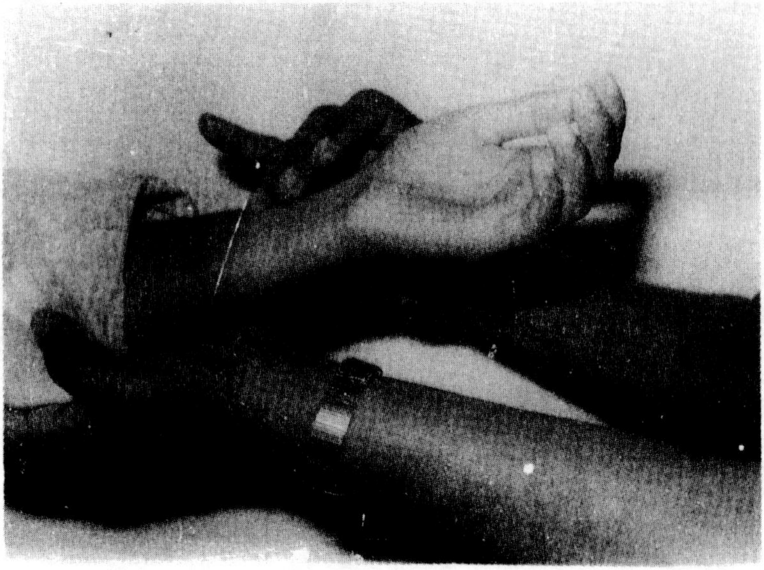

References

1. Relating to the Physician :

स्थिरचित्तो नीरोगश्च सुखासीनः प्रसन्नधीः ।
नाड़ी ज्ञान समर्थः स्यादित्याहुः परमर्षयः ।।
(नाड़ी ज्ञान तरंगिणी)

पीतमद्यश्चंचलात्मा मलमूत्रादि वेगयुत् ।
नाड़ी ज्ञानेऽसमर्थः स्याल्लोभाक्रान्तश्च-कामुकः ।।
(नाड़ी ज्ञान तरंगिणी)

स्थिरचित्तः प्रशान्तात्मा मनसा च विशारदः ।
ज्ञानार्थं रोगिणो वैद्यो निज दक्षिणपाणिना ।।
(योग रत्नाकर)

2. Relating to the Patients :

सद्यः स्नातस्य सुप्तस्य क्षुत्तृष्णातपशीलिनः ।
व्यायामश्रान्तदेहस्य सम्यग् नाड़ी न बुध्यते ।।
(भाव प्रकाश)

भुक्तस्य सद्यःस्नातस्य निद्रितस्योपवासिनः
व्यवायश्रान्त देहस्य भूतावेशिनि रोदने।
सुन्दरीणां च संयोगे मद्यपाने मतिभ्रमे
अपस्मारे श्रान्तदेहे नाड़ी सम्यग् न बुध्यते।।

(वसवराजीयम्)

त्यक्तमूत्र पुरीषस्य सुखासीनस्य रोगिणः।
अन्तर्जानू करस्यापि नाड़ी सम्यग् परीक्ष्येत्।।

(नाड़ी ज्ञान तरंगिणी)

3. Relating to Examination :

अंगुलिभिस्तु तिसृभिर्नाडीमवहितः स्पृशेत्। (भाव प्रकाश)
ईषाद्विनम्रकृत कूर्पर वामभागे
हस्ते प्रसारित सदंगुलि संधिकेय।
अंगुष्ठ मूल परिपश्चिम भागमध्ये
नाड़ी प्रभात समये प्रहरं परीक्ष्य।।

(योग रत्नाकर)

एकाङ्गुलं परित्यज्य मणिबन्धे परीक्षयेत्।
अधःकरेण निष्पीडय त्रिभिरङ्ग् गुलिभि भिर्मुहुः।।
लघुवामेन हस्तेन चालम्ब्यातुर कूर्परम्।।
स्फुरणं नाड़िकायास्तु शास्त्रेणानुभवैर्निजैः।।

(नाड़ी परीक्षा)

बार त्रयं परीक्षेत् धृत्वा धृत्वा विमोचयेत्।
विमृश्य बहुधा बुद्धया रोग व्यक्तिं विनिर्दिशेत्।।

(योग रत्नाकर)

प्रायः स्फुटा भवति वामकरे बधूनाम्।
पुंसां च दक्षिणकरे तदियं परीक्षा।।

(योगरत्नाकर)

Synonyms of Nadi

There is a great significance of synonyms in Ayurveda.

The book "Nadi Vigyan" written by Kanad and Yogaratnakar have following synonyms :

1. Jeevnadi — It tells us the position of Soul.
2. Snayu — Helps in cleaning the body.
3. Nadi — Being hollow.
4. Hansi — Being mobile itself, it also helps in movement of other organs.
5. Dhamani — Due to Palpation
6. Dhara — Helps in development of body
7. Dharani — Helps in maintenance of body.
8. Tantuki — Present everywhere in the body.
9. Jeevan Gyaana — Receiving knowledge of life through the Nadi.
10. Vasa — Covering the blood or having a smooth structure.
11. Hinshra — When disturbed causes death or death signals.
12. Dhaamani — Responsible for pulsation.
13. Jevitagya — Survival of a person is indicated by this nadi.
14. Jivsakshi — Showing the changes and different states in a living body.
15. Shira — Helps in blood circulation.
16. Sarvanga — Spread all over the body.
17. Jivatagya — Indicates the conditions of a living person.
18. Nadika — Being hollow.
19. Rasayani — Helps in circulation of blood fluids.
20. Nabj — 'Nadi' is called Nabj in Unani system.
21. Pulse — Modern medical science uses the word pulse for Nadi.

3

Sites of Pulse Examination

- अङ्गुष्ठमूलसंस्था तु विशेषेण परीक्ष्यते ।
  सा हि सर्वाङ्गगा नाड़ी पूर्वाचार्यैः सुभाषिता ।। (नाडी परीक्षा)
- पाणिपात्कण्ठनासाऽक्षि कर्णजिव्हा च मेढ्रगा । (वसवराजीयम्)
- वामदक्षिणतो लक्ष्याः षोडश प्राणप्रवोधकाः ।। (वसवराजीयम्)
- पाद्योर्नाडिकास्थाने गुल्फस्याधोऽङ्गुलिद्वयम् । (वैद्यभूषण)
- आगन्तुकं ज्वरं तृष्णामायासं मैथुनं क्लमम् ।
  भयं शोकं च कोपं च कण्ठनाड़ी विनिर्दिशेत् ।। (वसवराजीयम्)
- मरणं जीवनं कामं कण्ठरोगं शिरोरूजम् ।
  श्रवणानिलजान् रोगान् नासानाडी प्रकाशयेत् ।। (वसवराजीयम्)

The blood vessels are spread in each and every part and help in circulation of blood all over the body. Normally, the human heart contracts and relaxes at the rate of seventy two beats per minute and circulates blood all over the body. As a result pulsation is noticed in blood vessels. Arteries carry pure blood and are situated deep under the dermis. The veins carry impure blood from different parts of body and are superficial. Thus veins are always superficial but at certain regions even the arteries become superficial where their pulsation can be felt. Acharyas have thus described eight centres on both the sides of the body where the pulse can be examined.

Hands, legs, neck, nose-root, eyes-root, ears-root, tongue-root and penis-root are the places where the pulse can be examined.

1. Angusth Mool : The pulsation of Radial artery can be noticed at the base of the thumb. The above shlokas have described this 'Jeevanadi'. Examining the pulse at this position has become a routine practice due to various reasons.

2. Paad Mool (Gulf Prant) : Medically on the posterior part of the ankle joint (Gulf Sandhi) at a distance of two fingers 'Paad-Nadi' i.e. Posterior Tibial artery can be palpated. Some Acharyas have directed a three finger, while others have advised a two finger test for examining this pulse.

3. Karnamool (below the ears) : Posteriorly below the ear there is a small notch where the movement of posterior Auricular branch of External Carotid Artery is noticed. Only one finger is required to test the pulse at this place.

4. Greeva Mool (in the neck region) : On both sides of the throat are situated the Common Carotid Arteries hence the beats of these arteries are noticed in between the fibres of sternocleidomastoid muscle. By keeping only two fingers, a physician can examine the pulse. This pulse can be examined during Malarial fever, thirst, exertion, after exertion, after intercourse, during fear, depression and anger etc.

5. Nasa Mool : By keeping two fingers a physician can examine the pulse. Actually the Facial branch of the External Carotid artery is examined. Life-death, anxiety, throat problem, ear problem etc. can be known through this pulse.

6. Netra Nadi (pulse at the eye) : Beside the lateral canthus of the eye balls in the region above the cheeks, lies the Superficial Temporal artery. The pulse rate of this artery can be checked by using one finger. This artery can help us to know psychological condition, life and death.

7. Jeevha Mool : The movements of lingual branch of external carotid artery can be noticed below the tongue. This tells about the problem of nose, throat, mouth, life and death.

8. Medhra Mool : In males, at the root region of the penis and in females at the inguinal region the External Iliac artery and the superficial external pundendal artery can be palpated.

It tells us about diseases like diseasesed genito urinary tract, paraplegia, filaria etc.

4

The Importance of 'Jeev-Naadi'

-अस्ति प्रकोष्ठगा नाडी मध्ये काऽपि समाश्रिता।
जीवनाडीति सा प्रोक्ता नन्दिना तत्ववेदिना।।

(रावण)

Acharyas like Ravana have described the importance of 'Jeev-Nadi'. The Radial artery situated at the base of thumb is of utmost importance. In general the term pulse examination implies the examination of the pulse at the wrist for the following reasons.

1. It is very easy to examine.
2. This is a very apt region where a physician can keep his three fingers to check the three doshas of a patient. At other places physician is directed to use only one finger or two fingers to examine the pulse which does not fulfil the motto of pulse examination.
3. The pulse is quite superficial as it is not covered by fats, muscles or other blood vessels, hence the pulsation of the pulse is very clear.
4. Ayurveda system says that it is the region where all the diseases can be known while in other regions, knowledge of only a few diseases is possible.
5. If the patient is unconscious, sleeping, standing, sitting, weak, a woman, a child etc. even then pulse examination at the wrist is very easy.
6. Normally, this region remains uncovered hence the patient does not hesitate to show the pulse to the physician. Here the local temperature is in tune with the external environment.
7. The physician can get differential findings even by rotating or moving the pulse. The condition of the walls of the blood vessel can also be easily observed.
8. The physician can relax the patients hands by giving it a support of his hands. He can adjust the patient's hand at different positions.

9. This region is much more clean than other parts and the physician does not require apparatus or instruments for the pulse examination.
10. This pulse indicates the 'Arishta' (death indicating) symptoms of the patient much more clearly.
11. The pulses of both the hands can be examined simultaneously without any difficulty.
12. While examining this pulse the physician can also note the facial expression of the patient. The physician can also observe skin, eyes, voice, physique, tongue etc. described in the 'Ashta-Pariksha' (eight fold examination).
13. In cardiac diseases the change can be observed by uplifting the hands of the patient above the cardiac region.
14. A physician can correlate the blood pressure with the pulse rate of the patient.
15. If a physician has knowledge of palmistry then he can examine the palm of the patient while examining the pulse.

5

Sources of "Nadi Gyaana"

1. शास्त्रेण सम्प्रदायेन तथा स्वानुभवेन वै।
   परीक्षा रत्नवच्चास्या त्वभ्यासादेव जायते। (योगरत्नाकर)

2. स्फुरणं नाडिकायास्तु शास्त्रेणानुभवैर्निजैः।
   सम्प्रदायेन वा यत्नात्परीक्षेत् भिषक्तमः।। (रावण)

According to the texts there are three sources of knowledge about 'Nadi'.

1. Grantha Adhyayana (Shastra) - Study of texts.
2. Guru-Updesh (Sampradaya) - teacher.
3. Anubhav (Svanubhav) - personal experience.

1. Grantha Adhyayana :

The origin of Ayurveda is the vedic literature. It is for this reason that Ayurveda is considered as a part (Upaang) of Atharvaveda. Preservation positive health and cure of diseases are the twin objectives of Ayurveda. Clinical examination is an important factor for the fulfilment of above motto. The movement of the pulse of a healthy person is descrised in many 'Nadi-Granthas' and which also deals with the diagnosis of the patient as a part of 'Ashta Vidhi Pariksha' in which 'Nadi-Pariksha' occupies the first place. It is because of these reasons that the ancient literature has dealt with the science of pulse examination in detail. The texts of medieval period like 'Yog-Ratnakar, Sharangdhar, Vasavarajiyam, Bhavprakash' etc. devote separate chapters on Nadi-Pariksha . There are other books on pulse examination which are written in verses.

Some of the important ones are :

Nadi Vigyan	—	(Kanad Bhudhar & Harita)
Nadi Pariksha	—	(Ravana)
Nadi Gyaan Tarangini	—	(Shri Raghunath Prasad)

Nadi Darpan	—	(Shri Dutta Ram Choube)
Nadi Prakash	—	(Shri Govinda Acharya)
Nadi Gyaan Darpan	—	
Nadi Vivek	—	

Recent treatises on pulse examination include:-

Nadi Darshan	—	(Vd. Tarashankar Mishra)
Abhinav Nadi Tantra	—	(Vd. Vishwanath Dwivedi)
Nadi Vigyan (English)	—	(Vd. S. D. Upadhayay)

Books certainly offer theoretical knowledge about pulse examination. But the details and the ancient traditional language involved in this subject makes it difficult to acquire skill in this art. Mere theoretical knowledge will not bestow skill in this art.

2. Guru Updesh :

Getting practical knowledge under the careful guidance of the Guru (teacher) is the main source of knowledge of pulse examination, Physicians have accepted the fact of getting practical knowlege under the guidance of a master. The main hindrance in the pulse examination is that by mere indirect touch with help of the continous beats of the pulse a physician has to consider many aspects from the similar palpation. It is clear that the subject of pulse examination is intricate and difficult to understand. Experts always emphasize the minutest details to the students so that they have a very clear idea and knowledge about this subject. But modern world has seen the decline of Guru-Shishya tradition and so teachers are not able to give the complete knowledge of this subject. The famous schools like 'Atreya-Sampradaya' or 'Dhanvantari-Sampradaya' in ancient era, 'Varanasi Sampradaya' and the 'Vangeeya Sampradaya' in recent era are eclipsed. Skilled physicians like Pandit Satyanarayan Shastri who were ever ready to teach any curious student are no longer seen.

3. Sva-Anubhava :

The third foundation of this subject is one's own experience. Text gives us theoretical knowledge, a teacher gives us complete detailed knowledge and our own experience builds up confidence in the skill and fine tunes practical understanding. Continuous practice of pulse examination helps us to understand the minute movements of the pulse and also decide the nature of the disease and correlates it with other diseases. Testing the pulse with full concentration confirming it with other examinations and keeping this in memory and examining again and again on different patients is the means of 'Sva-Anubhava'. This means that with continuous studies and repeated efforts a person can acquire the skill. The knowledgeable subjects by the 'Naadi' are so vast that even after prolonged practice a physician is not able to decide on all subjects, certainly Sva-Anubhava is most useful to acquire skill in this art and Sva-Anubhava in the master key to perfection in the art of patient diagnosis.

6

Fundamentals of Pulse Examination

As said before the pulse examination is a highly developed and sepcialised part of clinical examination (Sparsh Pariksha). While analysing different contexts we come to know that we have to examine the pulsation, movement of pulse, nature, force and condition of blood vessel. The positive findings received from the above examination help in diagnosis. Each concept has specfic utility and is a different process of examination.

Sfuran Sthala (according to site) :

आदौ च वहते वातो मध्ये पित्तं तथैव च।
अन्ते च वहते श्लेष्मा नाडिकात्रप लक्षणम्।।

At a distance of 1 finger below the base of the thumb on the lateral side of wrist, the physician keeps his `index' 'middle' and `ring' fingers to study the movements of the pulse to find out the nature of the "Doshas". The physician can easily palpate the "Vaat, Pitta and Kapha" at the 'index' 'middle' and 'ring' fingers respectively.

A different view is expressed by Kanad in his book "Naadi Vigyan".

वाताधिका वहेन्मध्ये त्वग्रे वहति पित्तला।
अन्ते च वहते श्लेष्मा मिश्रिते मिश्रलक्षणा।
आदौ च वहते पित्तं मध्ये श्लेष्मा तथैव च।
अन्ते प्रभन्जनो ज्ञेयः सर्वशास्त्रविशारदैः।।

During the vitiation in Vaat, Pitta, Kapha the pulsation is predominantly seen in the 'middle' 'index' and 'ring' fingers respectively.

If two Doshas are percieved simultaneously then a mixed movement (at both the regions or at the junction of the two regions) is observed. According to others references the pulsation due to Vaat, Pitta and Kapha is seen in 'ring' index and middle fingers respectively.

On critical perusal, it is evident that only the order of Vaat, Pitta and Kapha is changed. Heart supplies blood through blood vessels to all parts of the body and the Doshas are carried along with it.

प्रतिरोगमिति कुध्दो रोगाधिष्ठानगामिनीः।
रसायनीः प्रपद्याशु दोषा देहे विकुर्वते।। (अ ० ह० नि० 1/23)
नहि वातं सिराः केचिन्न पित्तं केवलं तथा।
श्लेष्माणं वा वहन्त्येता अतः सर्ववहाः स्थिताः ।। (सु० शा० 7/17)

It is natural for "Laghu, (light) char (mobile) Vyavai Vaat" to remain in front then comes comparatively less "Guru (heavy), Drava (liquid), Sar," Pitta" and then third is "Guru (heavy), Pichhil (stickt, Abhishyandi (congestant) Kapha) Direct knowledge of pulse examination obtained in "Nadi-Pariksha" is more scientific and practical than as metioned in Nadi Vigyan.

Nadi Gati (according to pulse movement) :

The texts dealing with pulse examination have given a detailed description of movement of pulse. The contraction and relaxation of heart causes pulsation in the Nadi and we touch the pulse to examine it. According to Ayurvedic text flow of "Vyaan-Vayu" (type of Vaat which spreads all over the body) propels the circulation of blood and movement of pulse.

रसोयःस्वच्छतांयाति स तत्रैवावतिष्ठते।
ततो व्यानेन विक्षिप्तः कृत्स्नं देहं प्रपद्यते।।

(अ. ह. - सूत्र)

अङ्गुष्ठमूलभागे या धमनी जीवसाक्षिणी।
तच्चेष्ट्या सुखं दुःखं ज्ञेयं कायस्य पण्डितैः।।

(नाड़ी परीक्षा)

With regard to the movement of the pulse two theories are relatively important —

1) Sankhya sambandhi (rate),

2) Vishishta gati sambandhi (specific movement).

1) The theory of "Sankhya" (rate) describes the various rates of pulse. For example the high pulse rate is known by the "Chapalaa,

Vegvati, Druta, Chanchala, Teevra, Atichapalaa, Vegvahini, Sheeghraga etc. and those which reveal the low pulse rate are "Manda, Mandgamanaa, Mandagamini, Atimanda, Ksheenagati etc. Detailed description about the changes in pulse rate according to age is described in Ayurveda.

षष्ठ्या स्पंदास्तु मात्राभिः षट्द् पंचाशद्भवन्तिहि ।
शिशोः सद्यः प्रसूतस्य पंचाशत् तदनन्तरम् ।।
चत्वारिंशत्ततः स्पन्दा षट्द् त्रिंशत् यौवने ततः ।
प्रौढस्यैकोन त्रिशंत् स्यु वार्धक्ये ऽष्टौ च विशंतिः ।।

(भूघर)

During the ancient period there was a method to count the pulse rate. Now-a-days we count the pulse beat per minute. In Ayurveda the pulse rate per 'Pal' is mentioned. 2.5 'Pal' make a minute. Pulse rate is found to be different at different ages. In this regard the views of modern medical science and Ayurveda are similar.

Rate of pulse beat per minute according to Ayurveda

Age	Pulse beat in Pal	Pulse beat in minute
New born	56	140
Infant	50	125
Child	40	100
Young	36	90
Middle aged	29	72.5
Old	28	70
Very old	31	77.5

The pulse rate is a deciding factor in patients, suffering from typhoid fever and heart disease. During fever for even 1°. rise in temperature of body the pulse rate increases by 10. Fever results in an increased pulse rate. Similarly a decrease in pulse rate indicates impairment of heart functioning. When a person is asleep or at rest the pulse rate decreases, while work or exercise increase the pulse rate.

2. Vishishta gati (specific movement) :

Following examples describe the specific beats of the pulse according to the variation of Doshas.

वातोद्रेके गतिं कुर्याज्जलौका सर्पयोरिव।
पित्तोद्रेके तु सा नाड़ी काकमण्डूकयोर्गतिम्।
हंसस्येव कफोद्रेके गतिं पारावतस्य वा।।
(नाड़ी परीक्षा)

In this way following adjectives are used for the description of specific beats "Vishama, Sarala, Vakra, Riju" etc. The clear concepts of different conditions of the Doshas, to diagnose a disease, is very important for a physician. Definitely it is difficult to understand hence continous and long practice is required. That is why Acharyas have defined the beats by giving examples of various organisms.

Dosha/Disease	Type of beat	Example
Vaat	Vakra gati (zig zag movemnet)	Snake, Leech
Pitta	Chapala (Throbbing)	Crow, Frog
Kapha	Mandgamana (slow)	Swan, Sparrow
Vaata Pitta	Vakra	Snake
Kapha pitta	sometimes fast or sometimes slow	Lava Bird
Ajeerna (Indigestion)	Paritojada	Earthworm
Visuchika (Cholera)	Utplutya-utplutya	Frog
Asadhyata (Incurable)	Durbala, Manda (Weak, slow)	Like a dead snake

Acquiring a clear knowledge of beats and correlating it with other is the criterion of this science.

Sfuran (Pulsation) :

The "Vyan Vayu" and cardiac contractions are responsible for the circulation of blood which leads to pulse beats. Difference in force of flow of blood causes the difference in pulse beat. The difference of pulse beat ultimately tells about Dosha status and various diseases. Generally Sfuran (pulsation) and pulse movement are taken as same but there is a minute difference between the two. Pulse movement gives an account of the flow of the blood in waves while pulsation tells us about the local dilatation of blood vessels. Above idea is also expressed in the former shlokas. The dilatation of radial artery due to forceful flow of blood indicates pulsation. Different types of pulsation are found according to the blood flow. A physician should give a slight pressure on the pulse to know the 'Sfuran Bal' (pulsation force). Words such as 'Poorna' Rikta, Vishada, Sookshma, Prabala, Durbala" mentioned in 'Nadi Granthas' are used in this context.

Guna Pariksha (characteristics of pulse) :

In this process of pulse examination the most intricate part is the "Guna Pariksha". This is because in comparison to site or rate, the nature i. e. Laghu (light), Guru (heavy), Ruksha (dry), Snigdha (Smooth), Sthula (thick) Sheeta (cold), Ushna (hot) etc. are more difficult to understand. During the examination it becomes increasingly difficult to indentify the site (Sthala), specific movement (gati) and characteristics of the pulse. But from the diagnostic point of view the above criteria are useful and necessary in the diagnosis of a disease. It is helpful in knowing the etiology and psychological condition of a patient.

While examining the pulse a physician has to be more careful because while touching the pulse he has to even think of the aspects which cannot be determined by simply palpating the pulse. Above all, one cannot directly touch the pulse. The skin acts as an obstacle in the way. Repeated-keen observation is the key to success. When a physician acquires skill in examining the position, rate and nature of the pulse then and then alone he can correlate the findings with the nature of the disease, etiology, diet, psychological condition, progress of the disease and habit of the patient.

Test	Region and process	Utility
1. Sthala (site)	By keeping three fingers at the base of the thumb and assessing the state of the Vaat, Pitta and Kapha chronologically.	Helps in deciding the psycho-somatic constitution. The predominance of the Dosha at that moment and the prognosis of the disease.
2. Gati (rate & specific movement)	Counting the rate for 1 to 2 minutes and examining the specific waves in the pulse by keeping three fingers on the pulse.	In knowing the accumulation of Doeshas (sanchay), vitiation of the Doshas (Prakop), obstruction (Aawran) etc. Prognosis and diagnosis of specific disease.
3. Guna (nature)	The test must be carried out with total concentration by keeping the 3 fingers and giving a slight pressure on the pulse and then releasing it or by moving and rotating the pulse, the nature of the pulse can be assessed	In knowing the diet and habits of the patient, etio-pathology of disease, acute, sub acute, and chronic conditions, emotions and prognosis.

Methodology of 'Guna' Pariksha' and their uses :

Nadi Guna	Method/Procedure	Utility
1. Sheeta (cold)	Applying pressure for a while and finding the pulse to be comparatively colder than skin.	It indicates predominance of Kapha, presence of Aam, chronic cardiac disorders, indigestion, diarrhoea.
2. Ushna (hot)	Applying pressure for a while and finding the pulse to be comparatively hotter than skin.	It indicates predominance of pitta, fever, anger, anxiety, excitment, blood disorders.
3. Snigdha (unct-uous)	By applying the pressure the physician examines the smooth-ness of the pulse which touches the skin while palpating	It indicates obesity, Aam, diabetes, condition of excess 'Rasa'.
4. Ruksha (ununct-uous)	By applying the pressure the physician examines the rough-ness of the pulse which touches the skin during pulsation.	It indicates 'Dhatukshaya', anaemic, Vaaticdisorder, tuberculosis, after taking Rooksha Aahar. (Roughage diet) .
5. Sthoola (thick)	The pulse found thick while touching.	It indicates disorders of Aam, obesity, predominance of Kapha, constipation, alcohohims diabetes.
6. Tanu (thin)	The Pulse found thin while touching.	It indicates Vaatic disorders, bleeding disorders, tuberculosis, Dhatukshaya, other deficiency disorders and chronicdiseases.
7. Guru (heavy)	The pulse moves slowly but forcefully.	It indicates disorders of Aam, Saamavastha, early stages of diseases, blood disorders, after taking meals & during pregnancy.
8. Laghu (light)	The pulse moves hastely but with weak force.	It indicates proper digestion chronic fever, hunger, leucorrhoea.
9. Mridu (soft)	The pulse found soft to touch	It indicates disorders of vata, pitta and kaphaj diarrhoea,
10. Kathin (hard)	The pulse found hard to touch	It indicates atherosclerosis indigestion, chronic constiption, chronic Vattic disorders, leprosy etc.

7

Method of Palpation (Sparshan Vidhi)

वारत्रयं परीक्षेत् धृत्वा धृत्वा विमाचयेत् ।
विमृश्य बहुधा बुद्धया रोग व्यक्तिं विनिर्दिशेत्।।
(योग रत्नाकर)

स्पर्शनात् पीड़नात् ध्मातात्वेदनान्मर्दनादपि
तासु प्राणस्य संचारं प्रयत्नेन विशोधयेत्
(नाड़ी तंत्र)

The fingers kept on the pulse for examination should be lifted and kept again and again. If a difference in pulse beat occurs due to pressure of the physician's finger then lift the fingers again, allow the independent movement of the pulse. Repeat this at least three times. Sometimes by lifting two fingers or one finger a physician notices the difference in pulse beat and mode of filling. The Acharyas have instructed to examine carefully the pulse beat and then arrive at diagnosis.

During pulse examination light touch, slight pressure, more pressure should be applied. The pulse should be moved from left to right and vice versa or sometimes it must be left free for examining the mode of filling. Actually it depends on what the physician wants to know from pulse examination. 'Budhaya' and 'Prayatnena' which imply whether we want to check the regularity, irregularity, rate difference, difference in impulse, position of the pulse, force of the blood in vessel etc. The mode of pulsation varies accordingly. For example -- if one wants to check the 'Nadi Bal' then one has to apply pressure and if one wants to know condition of the pulse then one has to rotate it. The best thing to do is to check all aspects of the pulse to get better results. One should first decide the process of examination and carry it out accordingly. The findings obtained must be kept in mind and then correlated. If there is a slight area of doubt then one should wait for some time and then repeat the process. If required, the position of the patient's hands and body must be changed and then re-examined.

I. Naadi Bal :

"Balvati, Prabala, Sabala, Nirbala, Durbala," etc. are different terms mentioned about "Naadi Bal". The process of testing the Naadi Bal is as follows:

The three fingers should be kept on the pulse and pressed to the extent that the pulse stops beating. This decides "Naadi Bal". If the beating of the pulse stops by applying a sligh pressure then the pulse is weak and if a greater pressure is needed to stop the pulse beat then the pulse is said to be strong. There is another opinion that pressure must be applied through ring finger, the middle and index fingers kept free to know the pulsation. The reason is that, in the process the presence or absence of pulsation can be felt clearly by the index and middle fingers. By releasing the pressure from the ring finger one can feel the approaching impulse very clearly which indicates the "Naddi Bal".

II. Laya (rhythm):–

Sama, Sarala, Prasanna, Niyamita, Vishama, Vishamgamini, Trutika, Gatikautilya" etc. are used to define rhythm of beats. The pulse should be examined for a minute to study the mode of beat. Modern medical science studies the rhythm on the basis of regular or irregular pulse. Sudden increase or decrease in pulse rate, missing of pulse beat, increase or decrease in strength of the pulse indicates a disorder in rhythm. These disorders are of two types:

1. Regularly - irregular.
2. Irregularly - irregular.

Regularly - irregular:

Regularly irregular means an increase or decrease in pulse rate after every two to five minutes or the disappearance of an impulse after 20, 10 or 8 impulses, e.g ectopic beats at fixed interval.

Irregularly - irregular:

Irregularly - irregular means that there is increase or decrease in the beats only. Sometimes there is disappearance of an impulse after 4 or 8 impulses as in atrial fibrillation. It must be remembered that there is an increase in pulse beat during inspiration while there is a decrease during expiration. Normally arrhythmia is found in heart disease especially because of abnormality in sino-auricular node or 'conduction.' It is difficult to find out the irregularity in tachycardia on the other hand it is easy to find out the irregularity in bradycardia and so the patient should be allowed to lie down comfortably and given cardiac sedative and then examine the irregularity. Irregular heart beats can also be confirmed by E.C.G.

III. "Poornata" (volume):

Words such as "Sthoola, 'poorna,' 'apoorna,' 'rikta,' 'sukshma,' 'krisha' etc. are used to define the volume of the pulse. With each contraction of the heart blood flows through the blood vessels which generates impulse. By keeping the three fingers on the pulse the "Poornata" of the pulse should be tested during every impulse. If the blood is completely filled in the blood vessels then the touch is raised sharply. This is called "full pulse". But if the blood vessel is not completely filled then the touch is weak and smooth. Such a pulse is called 'small' or 'thready' pulse. The volume of pulse indicates many types of systemic diseases. In cardiac problems where the heart beat increases or the strength of contraction abnormally increases then there is also an exceptional rise in volume of the pulse. For example fever, hypertension, mental anxiety, anger, renal disorder, toxic condition and vitiation of Pitta etc. In diseases, which cause, a deficiency in blood, decrease in heart beat or contracting force there is a decrease in "Poornta". For example: weakness, dehydration, anaemia, cholera, vomiting, liver disorders, deficiency states, leucorrhoea etc.

An average volume is a mark of sound health. A very low volume indicates collapse or emergency.

While examining the "Naadi Poornata" one should also check the elasticity of the blood vessel. If the vessel is hard then the 'Poornata' cannot be examined properly. Normal artery alone can indicates or 'Apoornate' 'Poornata'.

Condition of blood vessel:

The condition of the blood vessel varies according to the age, (e.g. arteriosclerosis). Increase in cholesterol level also leads to changes like atherosclerosis.

Besides, anatomical, psychological changes lead to structural changes in blood vessel which is responsible for permanent changes in the pulse beat and nature of the pulse. The five ways discussed in the process in which we can confirm the condition of the pulse by

'Mardan' (moving the pulse in left ⇋ right direction). In old age the elasticity of the blood vessel is reduced and so they become hard. Also atherosclerosis leads to internal changes in artery because of which the blood vessel becomes thick and lumen is reduced. The pulses of such patients remain tubelike i.e. they do not flatten on pressure. As a result some aspects of the nature of pulse remain unknown.

For differential diagnosis the condition of the blood vessel must be examined and be co-related with other clinical findings.

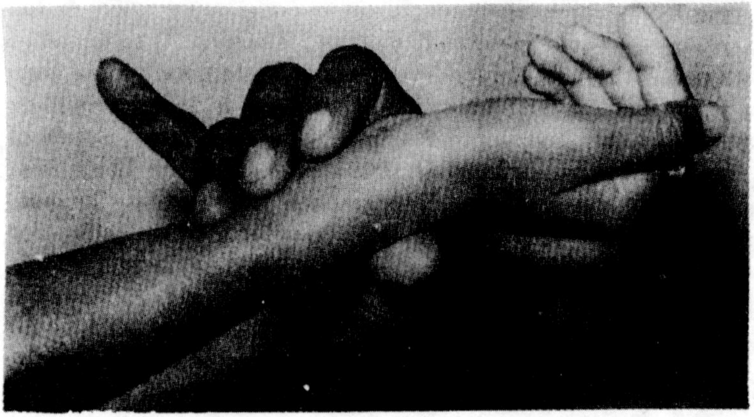

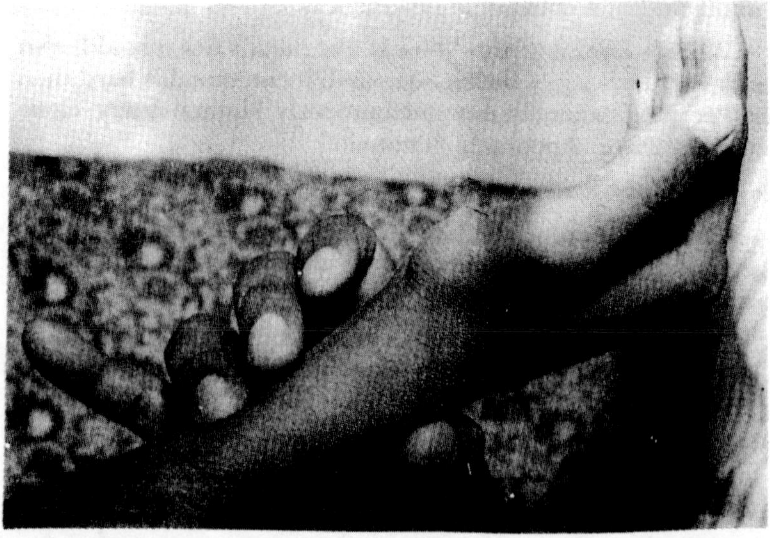

8

Doshas and Pulse Beat

The state of equillibrium and vitiation in the Doshas are responsible for health and disease respectively. There are three states of Doshas:

1. Vridhi (increase) 2. Kshaya (decrease) 3. Saamyataa (balanced condition)

"Saamyataa" indicates sound health of a person, while the 'Vridhi & Kshaya' are responsible for various ailments. Along with other physiological changes the pulse beat is also affected by these conditions.

दोषाः प्रवृद्धाः स्वंलिङ्गं दर्शयन्ति यथाबलम् ।
क्षीणाः जहति स्वं लिङ्गं समः स्वं कर्मकुर्वते ।।

i.e. increased Doshas enhance their functions while a decrease in Doshas decreases their functions while in normal condition they function normally. In the same way we get the state of the Doshas in the pulse i.e. during increased Doshas their predominance increases while a decrease in Doshas show a decrease in their conditional pulsation rate while in normal condition the Doshas are found in their respective regions and move at normal rate. As said before the predominance of Vata, Pitta and Kapha is seen below the 'index', 'middle' and the 'ring' fingers respectively.

वातेऽधिके भवेन्नाडी प्रव्यक्ता तर्जनीतले ।
पित्तेव्यक्ताऽथ मध्यायां तृतीयाङ्गुलिगा कफे ।।

The word 'Pravyaktataa' (predominance) means that the impulse can be noted below a certain finger with a greater vigour and without applying pressure. During this examination more attention must be given to the position of the fingers and the pressure of the finger, which means that the fingers should be kept in proper position and slight pressure must be given. By giving more pressure there can be a misunderstanding in the 'Pravyaktata' (predominance).

Knowledge of the Doshas according to pulse movement:

The specific movements according to the Doshas are mentioned in detail in Ayurveda. According to 'Gati Sankhya' (pulse rate) the 'Vaat Naadi' is found to be 'Vishama' i.e. it sometimes moves slowly while at times moves fast. The 'Pitta Naadi' is found to be 'Chapala' i.e. it moves fast while the 'Kapha Naadi' is found to be 'Sthira' i.e. it moves slowly.

वाते वक्रगतिर्नाड़ी चपला पित्तवाहिनी ।
स्थिरा श्लेष्मवती प्रोक्ता सर्वलिङ्.गा च सर्वगा ।
श्लेष्मगा स्तिमिता स्तब्धा मिश्रा मिश्रैस्तु लक्षयेत् ।। (नाड़ी परीक्षा)

Acharyas have described the specific movement of the pulse during a particular Doshic vitiation by giving various examples of the organisms. From the examples it is seen that the pulse movement are very minute. Another reason could be that even if different persons feel the same thing, their ways of expression may be different and hence by giving examples of the animals the Acharyas have given a clear way of understanding the pulse movement.

''वातोद्रेके गतिं कुर्यात् जलौकासर्पयोरिव ।
पित्तोद्रेके तु सा नाडी काकमण्डूकयोर्गतिम् ।
हंसस्येव कफोद्रेके गतिं पारावतस्य च ।। (अभिनव नाड़ीतंत्र)

Pulse according to different Doshas

Dosh	Sight at Naadi	Finger	Nature of Pulse Movement	Example	Modern view
Vata	Anterior	Index	Vakra	Snake Leech	Irregular
Pitta	Middle	Middle	Chanchal	Crow, Frog	Rapid
Kapha	Posterior	Ring	Mand	Swan, Pigeon	Slow
Pitta-Vata	Anterior-Middle	Index & Middle	Vakra Chanchal	Snake, frog (alternately)	Irregular +Rapid
Vata-Kapha	Anterior-posterior	Index -Ring	Vakra Manda	Snake Swan (alternately)	Irregular +Slow
Pitta-Kapha	Middle-Posterior	Middle & Ring	Sometimes Chanchal, sometimes Mand.	Frog, Peacock (alternately)	High Tension + slow
Tridosh	Whole region	Below the three fingers	Along with 'Vakra' Sometimes 'Teevra' Sometimes 'Mand'	Partridge Pheasant	Irregular +High tension +slow

9

Specific Movements

Due to the effect of the three 'Doshas' the mode of varies movement which has been described in various texts. Acharyas have defined them as 'Vakra, Chapalaa, Manda' etc. and have given examples of various animals to describe the same.

The extent of the doshas can be known by testing the pulse at the wrist on the basis of impulse, pulse-rate etc. The study of pulse movement is very critical and complex hence Acharyas felt the need to define it by giving examples of animals. If we look at the basic character of the Doshas then the change in pulse movement is very natural and logical but considering 'Jeevsakshinee-Naadi' as a mere blood vessel is not knowing the changes in pulsation, rate, position because of doshas. In fact changes do occur in blood vessels also. A change in emotions accounts for a change in blood pressure. Meals, places, hard work produce a profound effect on blood pressure which can be measured. Changes in blood pressure produce an effect on the blood vessel which can be experienced. As E.C.G., E.E.G., ultra sound, radio active isotopes are used to detect the disease. Similarly continuous practice of pulse examination can successfully be employed to know the type predominance of Doshas and extent of the disease. Apart from the pulse examination according to site, the specific movement can clearly indicate the doshic set up.

वाते वेक्रगतिर्नाड़ी पित्ताच्चपलगाभवेत् ।
कफान्मन्दगतिश्चैषा मिश्रिते मिश्रगाभवेत् ।। (नाड़ी ज्ञान तरंगिणी)

वाते वक्रगतिर्नाड़ी चपला पित्तवाहिनी ।।
स्थिरा श्लेष्मवती प्रोक्ता सर्वलिङ्गा च सर्वगा ।
श्लेष्मणा स्तिमिता स्तब्धा मिश्रा मिश्रैस्तु लक्षयेत् ।। (नाड़ी परीक्षा)

नाड़ीधत्ते मरूत्कोपे जलौकासर्पयोः गतिम् ।
कुलिंग काक मण्डूक गतिं पित्तस्य कोपतः ।
हंस पारावत गति धत्ते श्लेष्मप्रकोपतः ।।(शार्ङ्गधर संहिता)

Specific movement due to 'Vaat':-

अनृजु वातकोपेनं (नाड़ी तंत्र)

'Vakra, Vakragatika, Vishama etc. are the terms employed to define the pulse beat due to 'Vaat'. The word 'Vishama' is related to pulse rate' while 'Vakra' is related to the specific movement found in the pulse.

A physician must keep the three fingers on the pulse in a straight line and try to study the nature of beats. Whether the flow is in a straight line or in left/right direction or in a zig-zag manner e.g. movement of snake. This is 'Vakrataa'. Another type of 'Vakrataa' depends upon the irregular elevation of impulse. For example as in the case of leech where the beats may be high, moderate, low or sometimes very high. In my experience the type of 'Vakrataa' like a snake is found in Kapha-anu-bandh' and Kapha-anu-bandh Vaatic vitiation' and second type of 'Vakrataa' like a leech is found in 'Pitta-anu-bandh Vaatic vitiation'.

It may so happen that the impulse is observed only below one finger or two fingers. In this case also the nature of movement must be studied. At regions of 'Vaat' i.e. below the index finger if the above symptom or the 'Vakrataa' is seen then it is undoubtedly 'Vaatic' is disease.

वातिक नाड़ी

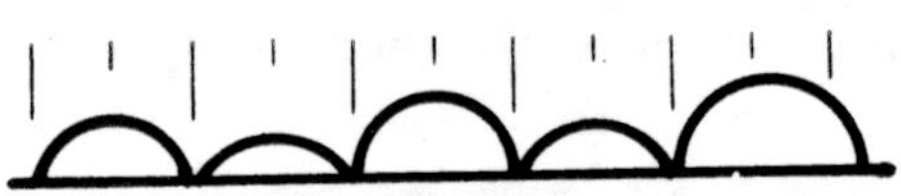

पित्तानुबन्धित वक्रगति
(जलौकावत्)

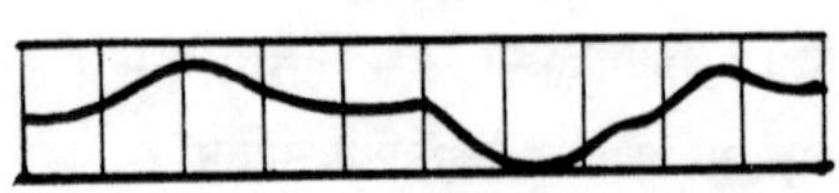

कफानुबन्धित वक्रगति
(सर्पवत्)

Movement of pulse due to 'Pitta' :-

चण्डा पित्तप्रकोपतः । (नाड़ी तंत्र)

'Chapalaa, Chapalgaa, Teevra' etc. are used to qualify the beats because of 'Pitta'. In this way both the increase in pulse rate and specific movement are possible due to 'Pitta'. Movement of animals such as crow, frog, sparrow etc. are used to describe 'pattic' movement. These animals leap while walking. This means there exists a gap when they jump from one place to another. Hence,'Pitta Naadi' has two basic features - height of impulse and interval between the two. From the above one can say that 'Pitta Nadi' has fast beat, high impulse and moves with an interval of space.

Kuling — Vaat-anubandh
Kaak — Vishudha-Pitta
Mandook — Kapha-anubandh

There can exist difference in pulse movement because of dosha-anubandh. Due to the effect of 'Vatanubandh' the beats observed are like a moving sparrow which are exceptionally fast, high but having small intervals. Due to vitiation of 'Pitta' alone the pulse movement is comparatively less fast with average interval like a moving crow. Due to Kapha-anubandh the beats are slow and the height of impulse increases gradually and then decreases suddenly and the interval is considerably large like a jumping frog.

Due to 'Vaat-Pitta' the blood vessels are thin.

पैत्तिक नाड़ी

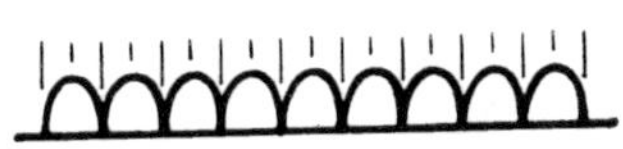

वातानुबान्धित (कुलिङ्गवत्)

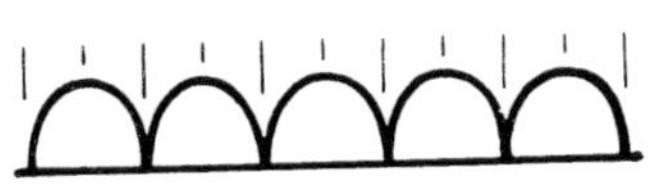

विशुध्द पित्त (काकवत्)

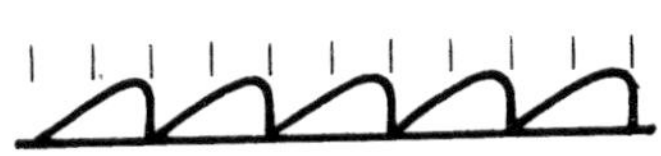

कफानुबान्धित (मण्डूकवत्)

Specific movement due to Kapha:

सरला.श्लेष्मकोपेन (नाड़ी तंत्र)
स्थिरा श्लेष्मवती प्रोक्ता सर्वलिङ्ग गाच सर्वगा ।
श्लेष्मणा स्तिमिता स्तब्धा मिश्रा मिश्रैस्तु लक्षयेत् ।। (नाड़ी परीक्षा)

Sthira, Stimita, Stabdha, Prasanna, etc. are the words employed to describe this pulse. 'Sthira and Stabdha' indicate a decrease in pulse rate. Viscosity & stickness can be noticed not only in Kapha but also in Aam (indigestion) and other Kapha-Vitiation.

'Prasanna' means that the pulse moves in full volume and in a regular rhythm.

Movent of animals such as swan, pegeon, elephant are used to give examples of specific movements. These animals walk in a steady manner without haste. Because of Kapha the pulse moves in continuous manner. In my opinion, a pulse moves in full volume regularly but slowly because of the Vaat-anu-bandh like a swan. It is 'Niyamita and Prasanna' but comparatively fast because of 'Pitta-annbandha' like Pigeon, Movements like an intoxicated elephant, such as 'Niyamita; Poorna, Sthula' but slow are alone because of Kapha. Due to Kapha the blood vessels are thick.

श्लैष्मिक नाड़ी

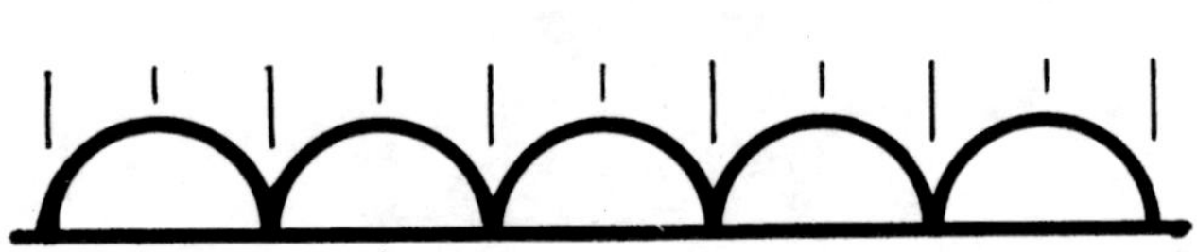

पित्तानुबन्ध (हँसवत्)

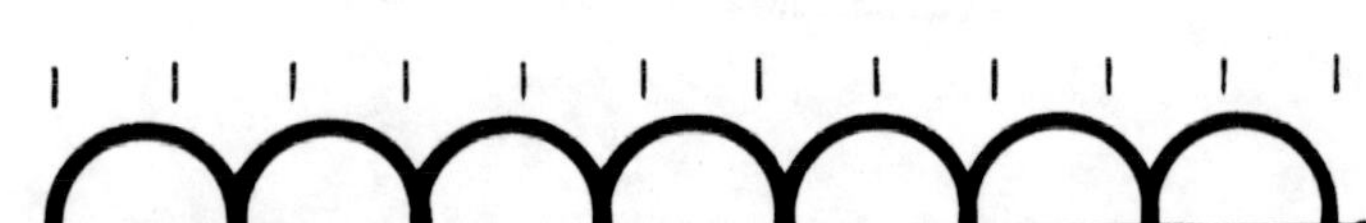

वातानुबन्ध (पारावत)

Dvandvaj & Sannipaatik Naadi:

नाड़ी धत्ते त्रिदोषे तु गतिं तित्तिरलावयोः ।
कदाचिन्मन्दगा नाड़ी कदाचिद्वेगवाहिनी ।।
दोषेद्वयोद्भवे रोगे विज्ञेया सा भिषग्वरैः ।। (नाड़ी परीक्षा)

The action of any two vitiated doshas or the ailments occurring due to them result in the respective specific movement of the pulse i.e. the pulse is found to possess the symptoms of both the vitiated dosha and the predominance is even observed in the respective region.

During the condition of 'Dvandaj Prakop', two theories are accepted. According to one of the theories, the symptoms of the two vitiated doshas are seen alternately. During the 'Vaatpitta Prakop' one observes the symptoms of 'Vaat' while at other times a 'Pitta Nadi' is observed. In fact the pulse movement changes according to the strength of Vitiated dosha.

According to another theory, during the vitiation of two doshas it is observed that at a particular doshic region, the symptoms of the other vitiated dosha are seen. For example:during 'Vaat-Kapha prakop' at the Kapha region, below the ring finger, one observes a 'Vakragati' i.e. symptom of Vata. Even in this case the strength of the vitiated dosha determines the nature of pulse and the region of predominance.

The nature of pulse during Sannipaatic Prakop' has been discussed in detail in various 'Naadi granthas'. Irregular rythms are the main symptoms of Sannipat (Tridosha vitiation).

कदाचिन्मन्दगा नाड़ी कदाचित् शीघ्रगा भवेत् ।
त्रिदोषप्रभवे नाड़ी विज्ञेया हि भिषग्वरैः (अभिनव नाड़ी तंत्र)

Acharyas have given examples of partridge, sparrow (which sometimes move, very fast while momentarily stops while walking) to define Tridoshic vitiation. Another example movement of the beak of the wood pecker, is also available. The 'Sannipat-Naadi' can clearly be felt below all the three fingers.

अंगुलित्रितयेऽपि स्यात् प्रव्यक्ता सन्निपाततः । (नाड़ी परीक्षा)
लाव-तित्तिर-वार्ताकगमनं सन्निपाततः । (अभिनव नाड़ी तंत्र)

Acharyas believe that during 'Sannipaat' the pulse beats are found to be fast flow or zig-zag below any of the fingers. In fact "uncertainty" is the characteristic of 'Tridosh Nadi' which can be found in site, rate, movement, strength, pulsation, temperature and condition of arterial walls.

10

Effect of 'Agni' on Pulse

'Agni' has been described as the basis of health. The whole body is affected by Agni so it naturally affects the pulse.

Angi and meals always affect the pulse. 'Mandaagni' results in indigestion of food which causes various types of 'ajeerna', 'ama', 'Vidhagdha', i.e., 'Vishtabdha', 'Rasashesha' and 'Dinpaaki' which the acharyas have defined as 'Roganikasya te moolam ajeernam propnuvanti hi'. A pulse moves slowly because of 'Aam' and due to 'Ajeerna' there is a deposition of materials on the inner walls of the blood vessels which results in the hardening of the blood vessel, hence they are hard and thick.

- लघ्वी वहति दीप्ताग्नेस्तथा वेगवती मता । (नाड़ी परीक्षा)

- सम्मूर्च्छनाद्यैर्जठराग्निमांद्यान्नाड़ी वहेत्तन्तुचला च जन्तोः । (नाड़ी परीक्षा)

During 'Deeptagni' the pulse is 'laghu' (light) and moves fast. In this case the digestion is proper, formation of 'Rasa' is also normal, hence the pulse is 'laghu' (light). The converse happens in 'Mandaagni' where the pulse is Guru (heavy), moves comparatively slowly. If 'Mandaagni' persists for a longer period of time the pulse beats are 'Kathina (hard), Jada, Tantuchala (thin). If 'Rasasheshajeerna', occurs then the pulse is found to be 'Sthula' (filled & thick) and moves fast. Rasasheshajeerna is the type of Ajeerna in which there is no desire to eat.

अजीर्णे तु भवेन्नाडी कठिना परितो जडा ।
चपला रसजे दीर्घा पित्ते वेगवती तथा ।। (नाड़ी परीक्षा)

One observes a 'Chapala Naadi' which is opposite of 'Jada Naa .i' in Annajeerna'. Shushrut says that the vitiations of the doshas increase because of 'Ajeerna' -- 'Ajeernat Pavanadinaam vibhramo Balvan Bhavet'. That is why the beats found below the three fingers vary. Acharyas call it as 'Parito Jada' and 'Deergha'. Due to persistant 'Ajeerna' the internal tissue state declines ('dhatukshay') resulting in a weak pulse with low tension.

पक्वाजीर्णे पुष्टिहीना मन्दं मन्दं वहेत्‌शिरा। (अभिनव नाड़ीतन्त्रे)

The differentiation of 'Saddyo Jeerna and Jeernajeerna' depends on the specific movements of the pulse. It is very necessary to understand the various movements and effect of Agni on pulse especially in abnormalities related to digestion.

11

Effect of Diet on the Pulse

Diets are not only the medium in building our body but are also necessary for physiological functions. A balanced diet is responsible for a healthy body while an unbalanced diet results in ailments. Diet effects the whole body including the pulse. The texts have depicted the effect of various types of diet on the pulse rate. Recent experimental evidence suggests that specific diet directly affects the pulse rate.

Effect of appetite on the pulse

चपला क्षुधितस्य स्यात्। (नाड़ी परीक्षा)

प्रसन्ना च द्रुता शीघ्रा क्षुद्भिर्नाडी प्रवर्त्तते। (नाड़ी परीक्षा)

The beats of hungry individual are fast. If by any means man does not get food for a day then the pulse declines, grows weak, becomes empty and contracts, the pulsation is dominated by Vata or Pitta. That is why, testing the pulse of a hungry man is not advised because it does not give the real physical state of the pulse and hence failure to detect the body condition.

Pulse beat after meals :

स्थिरा तृप्तस्य सा भवेत् । (नाड़ी परीक्षा)

कफवत् तृप्त दृप्तयोः। (नाड़ी परीक्षा)

After meals the beats of pulse are found to be slow (sthira). According to the doctrine of Ayurveda there is an increase of Kapha after meals and hence the beats after the meals are mainly dominated by Kapha. The pulse rate will be comparatively low and the pulse will be 'Poorna (full). Prasanna and Balayukta in force. The flow of blood after the meals is more towards the digestive system hence there is a marked decrease in the amount of blood flowing towards the brain and that is why one feels lazy and drowsy. Due to this the work of 'Vagus nerve' which controls the cardiac beat; declines and this ultimately decrease the heart beat. With the process of digestion there is a marked increase in quantity of blood especially the plasma fluids, hence the Nadi remains as 'Prasanna and Poorna'.

Due to this effect of meals the pulse rate does not indicate the true physical state of the body, hence the pulse should not be examined immediately after meals.

Effect of various 'Rasas' on pulse

Ayurveda has described six Rasas which have a direct relationship with the doshas. Some of them are 'Prakopak' (causing excitation) while others are Prashaamak (causing sedation) of doshas.

Dosha	Prakopak Rasa	Prashaamak Rasa
Vata	Kashaya, Katu, Tikta	Madhur, Amla, Lavana
Pitta	Amla, Katu, Lavana	Madhur, Tikta, Kashaya
Kapha	Madhur, Amla, Lavana	Katu, Tikta, Kashaya

Meals are more taste based while medicines mainly contain active principals. An increase or decrease in the doshas takes place according to the nature of diet. Thus the pulse rate also varies accordingly. One thing has to be remembered that the assimilation, effect, spread of the doshas cannot be sighted immediately but diets do have an immediate effect on the nature of pulse beat which can be experienced. For example after an intake of sweet and salty diet as the 'Guru guna' (heaviness) increases, the nature of pulse is 'Sarala'. (steady).

Effect of 'Madhur Rasa' on the pulse :

मधुरे बहिर्गानाड़ी (कणाद)

मधुरे हँसगामिनी (नाड़ी ज्ञान तरंगिणी)

'Madhur Rasa' originates from the 'Prithavi and Jala Mahabhootas, hence increases the Kapha in our body. So prolonged intake of 'Madhur Rasa' results in slow, outwardly beats, prominent in the region of 'Kapha. These changes are permanent in persons habituated to diet with 'Madhur Rasa'. It is natural that there is an increase in Kapha after the meals but with the intake of 'Madhur Rasa' the 'Rasa Kapha' increases sharply, so the symptoms of Kapha are mainly found after the intake of 'Madhur Rasa'.

Effect of 'Amla Rasa' on the pulse :

1. अम्ले कोष्णा प्लवगतिः। (कणाद)

2. अम्ले भेक गतिः कोष्णा। (नाड़ी ज्ञान तरंगिणी)

The 'Amla Rasa' increases the 'Pitta' and represents the 'Prithavi and Agna Mahabhootas'. The habitual or prolonged intake of 'Amla Rasa' results in leaping of pulse, slightly hot to touch. The specific movement of the pulse resembles the movements of frog with the pre-dominance of 'Pitta' in the persons taking 'Amla Rasa'. The pulse is more obvious at the 'Pitta' region but the qualities such as thin, swiftness associated with 'Pitta' will not be observed or will be minimun. It must be remembered that during digestion, (Paripaak Kaal) the predominance of 'Pitta' is also observed. So we must be careful about differences existing in the above pulses on the basis of behaviour and pulse exaination after food intake.

Effect of 'Madhur-Amla Rasa' on the pulse :

1. अम्लैश्च मधुराम्लैश्च नाड़ी शीता विशेषतः। (कणाद)
2. द्रव्यैश्च मधुराम्लाद्यैर्नाडी शीता विशेषतः। (नाड़ी ज्ञान तरंगिणी)

With the intake of many things dominated by 'Amla Rasa', Madhur Rasa or Amla-Madhur Rasa' then apart from above symptoms the pulse is also found to be cold.

Effect of 'Lavan a Rasa' on the pulse :

लवणे सरला द्रुता। (कणाद)

'Lavana Rasa' has more of 'Jal and Agni' in terms of the 'Panch mahabhootas' and thus increases the 'Pitta and Kapha' simultaneously, hence with the intake of 'Lavana Rasa' the pulse moves swiftly in a straight direction. The increase in rate is due to 'Pitta' while Kapha imparts a directional character to its movements. The pulse of such a person is 'Poorna' and possesses an average strength. From the point of nature of the pulse, it is found to be smooth, soft, heavy, sometimes hot and sometimes cold. It is more obvious in the region of 'Kapha and Pitta'.

Effect of 'Katu Rasa' on the pulse :

1. कटुके भृंग सन्निभाः। (कणाद)
2. चपला कटुकादेश्च भक्षणात्।। (नाड़ी विज्ञान)

The 'Katu Rasa' originates from 'Vayu and Agni'. This Rasa causes an increase in Vata & Pitta. The movement of the pulse is like a large black bee i.e. the rate is very fast but the pulsation area is less which means that the pulse seems to move fast in the middle of 'Vaat-Pitta' region. The pulse is soft and 'Ushna-Laghu' (hot & light).

Effect of 'Tikta Rasa' on the pulse :

1. तिक्ते स्याद भूलतागतिः । (कणाद)

2. तिक्ते स्थूल गतिर्भवेत् । (नाड़ी ज्ञान तरंगिणी)

The basis of 'Tikta Rasa' is 'Vayu and Aakash' in terms of 'Panchmahabhootas', hence with the intake there is an increase in 'Vayu'. The pulse moves like an earthworm i.e. pulse rate will be slow but it would follow a curved movement. The pulse is thick.

Effect of 'Kashaya Rasa' on the pulse :

कषाये कठिना म्लाना। (कणाद)

The origin of this Rasa is 'Prithivi and Vayu' in terms of 'Panchmahabhootas' hence it increases 'Vaat'. With habitual or prolonged intake of this Rasa the pulse is found to be hard with a low rate. 'Kashaya Rasa' is contractive, adds viscosity and reduces the flow of blood, hence the pulse is hard to touch and the pulse rate also decreases. It is more clear in the region of 'Vata.

Effect of two or three 'Rasas', on the pulse :

एवं द्वित्रि चतुर्योगे नानाधर्मवती धरा। (नाड़ी ज्ञान तरंगिणी)

If a person takes two or three or four 'Rasas' simultaneously then from above, the pulse movement will be expressive of various effects alternatively or will be simultaneous. If one notices different types of beats then one should understand that the patient has taken different 'Rasas' at one time.

Effect of specific meals on pulse :

The texts describe various meals which produce specific effects on the pulse rate. On thinking over the different examples one finds that there is a certain relation between the pulse rate and diet according to the doshas or quality of diet but some types of beats cannot be related with the nature of the diet. This is perhaps because of the specific effect of the specific diet which leads to the specific types of pulse beats. Some important meals and their various pulse movements are described.

1. निरन्तरं खरं रूक्षमन्नमश्नाति वातलम्।

रूक्षा वातोल्बणा तस्य नाड़ी स्यात्पिण्ड़सन्निभा।। (नाड़ी विज्ञान)

2. रूक्षे शुष्के च अल्पे च भोजने नाड़िका गतिः।

चपला त्वरिता हीना कृशाङ्गी चैव दुर्बला।। (अभिनव नाड़ी तन्त्र)

'Khar', (rough), Rooksha, (ununctuoua), 'Shushka' (dry), Vaatvardhaka continuous light diet (low nutrition diet) makes the pulse 'Rooksha' (rough) swift, Apporna (partially filled) thin, narrow and weak. Disease caused by malnutrition also has the same effect on the pulse. Such a pulse is also found in dehydration, anaemia and chronic diseases.

With the intake of high caloric diet, fried foods, foods made with jaggery, non-veg food, food made up of milk, maida etc., the pulse is found to be slow and moving orderly in its own position in fixed direction. It is hard to touch comparatively, cold and forceful. To express such movement Acharyas have used words 'Hansvat, Stimitvega, Sthirvaha, Sthira, Manda,' etc. All these are high caloric diets providing instant energy and hence the pulse possesses 'Poornataa', completely filled up and moves forcefully.

1. रम्भागुडवटाहारे माषद्विदलनिर्मिते।

गंभीरगतिः सा स्याद् गुर्वी व लगुडाकृतिः।।

(अभिनव नाड़ी तन्त्र)

2. पुष्टिगोधूमचूर्णेन घृतनिर्मितभोजनात्।

नाडी स्थिरा मन्दा च गुर्वी सामा गरीयसी।।

(अभिनव नाड़ी तन्त्र)

As said before, with the intake of high caloric foodstuff made up of jaggery, urad dal, flour, ghee and bananas, the pulse is found to have comparatively slow movement. It moves in its position with heavy and 'Saam gati'. Due to these high caloric diets the pulse at the Kapha region is more obvious but if 'Tikta, Katu and Amla Rasa' are also included then the pulse is found sluggish in the 'vaat-pitta' region.

गुड–रंभा–मांससौहित्य कटुतीक्ष्णाम्लभोजनैः।

वातपित्तार्तिरूपेण नाड़ी वहति निश्चला।। (अभिनव नाड़ी तन्त्र)

Apart from this with the intake of things such as white gourd, raddish, the pulse moves slowly. With intake of leafy vegetable the pulse moves with full volume and is warm to touch. Things such as salty mixture (Chivda) and roasted gram when taken along with curd or milk give a sluggish movement to the pulse. With the intake of excess liquid diet the pulse assumes full volume, moves slowly and cold to touch. With intake of liquids and solids simultaneously the pulse may be sometimes hard or soft to touch. The pulse becomes full in volume and moves slowly with the intake of butter milk.

But if it is sour or is taken in large quantities then the pulse becomes 'Vyakula' i.e. it may sometimes be fast or slow in its movement. Citrus food such as lemon, sweet lime, oranges, pomegranates etc. make the pulse 'Prasanna, Laghu & fast in its movements.

1. शर्करादधिसंयुक्तां मथितां द्रवपानतः।
   नाड़ी प्रसन्ना गम्भीरा भवेत् सा मंदगामिनी।।
   तदैवाधिकापानेन व्याकुला पुष्टिदातु सा। (अभिनव नाड़ी तन्त्र)

2. कर्कटीनागरंगे च दाडिमाम्लरसग्रहे।
   भवेत् प्रसन्ना लघ्वी तथा द्रुततरा गतिः।। (अभिनव नाड़ी तन्त्र)

Popular cold drinks also are included in these but as they contain certain chemicals, they make the pulse 'laghu' and the pulse moves fast in the region of 'Pitta'. But drinks such as Cola in which there is effervescence, effect is promounced the region of 'Vata'. It is also necessary to mention the popular stimulant, such as tea or coffee. From our very personal experience we feel that the pulse becomes warm and moves fast in the region of 'Pitta'. Normally patients come in the morning having their cup of tea and so it becomes very difficult to study the pulse, hence during examination the intake of tea must also be accounted.

Effect of Vihar (phycical movement) on the pulse beat :

Some specific physical movements do create profound effect on the pulse. Acharyas have described such 'Vihar' and their respective effects on pulse. Some create an immediate and temporary effect while others prolonged and habituated 'Viharas' produce permanent effect on the pulse. For example when a person runs, then there is sudden increase in pulse rate but for athelete runners the pulse is found to be moving slowly.

व्यायामे भ्रमणाच्चैव चिन्तायां धनशोकतः।
नाना प्रकार गमना जीवितज्ञा भवेद् ध्रुवम्।।

(नाड़ी ज्ञान तरंगिणी)

Due to exercise and journey the pulse does not remain the same, infact, it goes on changing. Acharya Ravana says that because of over exertion the pulse beats are found to be missing. After exertion the pulse is found to be weak. Pulse should not be examined after bath as the pulse moves with 'Manthar gati' (slow movement) and is found to be thready.

रिरंसोरूज्झितरतेश्चलतोऽपि च वातवत्।

(नाड़ी परीक्षा)

The pulse of persons with lust or desires for sex, after intercourse or walking moves like 'Vaat Naadi' i. e. the pulse becomes 'Alpa, Teevra, Vakragati, Rooksha and Laghu'. According to 'Naadi Gyaan Tarangini' pulse of a person after intercourse moves fast and in straight direction.

मैथुनान्ते भवेच्छीघ्रा सरलापि च नाड़िका।

The pulse of a lazy person or a person during sleep and willing to sleep, moves like a kapha Naadi' i. e. it is full in volume and moves slowly.

निद्रालोः .... कफवत्। (नाड़ी विज्ञान)

The pulse of a person who wakes for the whole night moves erraticaly with excitedness like a 'Vaat Naadi'. During suppression of excretory urges (Adharniya veg) the pulse moves like 'Pitta Naadi' i. e. it moves fast with leaps and is found to be hot.

रूद्धवेगस्य .... पित्तवत्। (नाड़ी विज्ञान)

The pulse of a person going on journey or returning back from a journey is also found to be of various types and so it is not constant.

It is because of these reasons that Acharyas have advised, not to check the pulse of a person who has just taken a bath , had meals, who is tired with exercise, had an intercourse, returned from journey. If it becomes necessary to examine the pulse then the examination must be done with great care and concentration. Only after this the state of a patient can be assessed.

एतेषां नाड़िका वैद्यो प्रयत्नेन विलोकयेत्।
सम्यग – ज्ञात्वा ततो नाड़ीं सर्वं वाच्यं शुभाशुभम्।
(नाड़ी विज्ञान)

Effect of emotions on the pulse :

Ayurveda has given a detailed description about the 'Mana' (mind) Atma (soul and Sharir (body) which constitute the tripod of living organism and the whole life depends on them. Of the three, 'Mana' is very important. The psycological condition certainly affects the physical state of a person.

The psychological emotions produce a direct and immediate effect on the body, especially the nervous system and the circulatory system. The face turns red during anger and pale during fear. During anger, excitedness, lust there is greater secretion of stimulating neuroharmones such as adrenaline, nor adrenaline which ultimately increase the heart beat and the pulse rate. During the state of fear or depression, 'depressant' such as acetylcholine is excessively secreted that leads to slow pulse rate and blood circulation. Hence the pulse is found to be weak.

According to Acharya Sharangdhar the pulse beat is fast during anger or lust while it is slow during depresion.

काम क्रोधात् वेगवहा, क्षीणा चिन्ता भयप्लुता। (शार्ङ्गधर संहिता)

According to Acharya Ravana the pulse moves weakly (Ksheena) during excitedness, anger, lust, ' ~sion or fear.

उद्वेगक्रोधकामेषु भयचिन्तोदये तथा।
भवेत्क्षीणगतिर्नाडी ज्ञातव्या वैद्यसत्तमैः।।
(नाड़ी परीक्षा)

From the above examples there is a difference in opinions. If we take it from the 'effect of disease' point of view then we find that there is a difference only in words but the meaning is same.

काम शोकभयात् वायुः क्रोधात् पित्तं त्रयोमलाः।
भूताभिषंगात् कुप्यन्ति दोष सामान्य लक्षणः।।
(माधव निदान)

'Vata' increases with the effect of lust, sorrow, fear hence the beat of the pulse vary from slow to fast or irregular. 'Ksheena' means that it becomes weak in force. Pitta increases with anger hence the pulse movements are fast and is hot to touch but after anger subsides, it is found to be weak and slow. In the above context the pulse movement varies pare due to tension, sorrow, or loss of wealth. The pulse of a person full of hatred is found to be unstable i.e. it may sometimes be slow or fast. It may be weak while at times be strong. The pulse of a person living a happy and contented life is found to be stable.

सुखेरतस्य शिथिलं प्रयाति। (अभिनव नाड़ी तन्त्र)

In the 'Sadhya-a-sadhya' (curable or incurable) chapter we find that emotions such as fear, sorrow etc. are the main reasons by which even a deeply feeble pulse does not indicate bad prognosis and because of sorrow, it does not move in its position i.e. it gets displaced and is inert but this does not indicate bad prognosis.

भारप्रवाहमूर्च्छाभयशोकप्रमुखकारणान्नाडी।
संम्मूर्च्छिताऽपि गाढं पुनरपि सा जीवितं भजते।। (नाड़ी परीक्षा)
स्वस्थानहीना शोके च हिमाक्रान्ते च निर्गदाः।
भवन्ति निश्चला नाड्यो न किंचित् तत्र वै भयम्।। (अभिनव नाड़ी तन्त्र)

With the sudden shock of fear or sorrow we get a missed beat, displaced and cold pulse. It should not be considered as an indication of bad prognosis.

The pulse of an excited or a crazy person sometimes shows the predominance of one dosha, two doshas or perhaps three doshas.

उन्मत्तानामभिचार विमूढ़ मनसामपि।
व्यस्तं, समस्तं, द्वन्दं च दोष रूप विशेषतः।। (कणाद)

The effect of emotional state is temporary, as the mental condition changes there is a change in the nature of pulse also. There is a permanent change in pulse in case of a psychic ailment. The diagnosis should be carefully done by correlating the mental-physical symptoms and the effect of mental condition on the pulse.

12

Diseases and Pulse-beat

Diagnosis of disease is the basic aim of patient's examination. The various texts have discribed the different pulse beats according to the disease. Many physicians diagnose the disease by pulse examination.

रुजाकालिक वैशिष्ट्यात् भवेत्सापि विलक्षणा। (अभिनव नाड़ी तंत्र)

Pulse beat varies according to the diseases and the various stages of the diseases.

'Rogastu dosho vaishamyam' -

Imbalance of doshas lead to disease according to the 'Shloka'. The detection of pulse beat according to the doshas helps knowing at the disease. Since human body is made up of large collection of living cells, certain biochemical changes continuously take place in the body. Because of this reason there is a difference in pathogenesis. Hence sometimes we can diagnose the disease according to dosha while at times we can find an appreciable difference in it. Acharyas have defined the above two conditions as 'Prakriti sam samvaya' and 'Vikriti visham samvaya'. It means that in 'Prakriti sam samvaya' we get the pulse beat according to the doshas while in 'Vikriti visham samvaya' we find a different pulse beat irrespective of doshas.

Above all, the 'Kaaran, Aashraya, Shrotas, Rogmarg, Agni and Vyadhi bal etc. have their various effects on the pulse in various disorders.

It is clear that the beats according to the disease do have a practical and theoretical support. Logical scientific reasons and minute clinical observation of Acharyas confirm the same.

A clinician having a clear concept of the pulse beat will be skilled in the art of diagnosis.

The pulses according to the diseases are described below :

Pulse during fever :

- उष्णा वेगवती नाड़ी ज्वरकोपे प्रजायते। (नाड़ी परीक्षा)
- ज्वरकोपे तु धमनी सोष्णा वेगवती भवेत्। (नाड़ी परीक्षा)

The pulse beat increases during fever and the skin along with the pulse is hot to touch. If a patient tends to sweat and is sitting in open air then even in fever the skin is found to be cold but when the pulse is pressed with pressure then we can find that it is hot. By examining the pulse in this way we can get the right information about 'Mandajvara (mild fever), Dhatujvara, Vishamajvara (malaria), Rajayakshama (T. B.) etc. Patient having 'Angamard (body ache), Mukhvraiasya (tastelessness) Klum (fatigue)', along with hot and increased pulse rate, when given proper medicine gives miraculous response. Our normal body temperature is 36^0 C or 98.4^0 F. and our pulse rate is 72 beats per minute. With every rise in 1^0. there is a rise of 10 beats per minute. This is due to increase in body temperature which increases the heart beat, hence it is easy to find out rise in temperature. This practice of examining the pulse is followed by each and every physician.

Pulse beat before fever (predisposing stage of fever) :

The pulse can give the knowledge about the pre-clinical condition of fever. With the increasing temperature there is a corresponding increase in pulse rate but during the condition before fever the temperature of the body is less, hence we do not find a marked increase in the pulse beat but the pulse beat is found to be expanded and hot to touch.

ज्वरे तीव्रा प्रसन्ना च नाड़ी वहति पित्ततः । (नाड़ी परीक्षा)

Here 'Prasanna' means without any abnormality or load. These symptoms are clearly found during the increase of 'Pitta' but 'Prasanna' may not be found during fever or before fever and during Saam (with Aam) or Niraam (without Aam) conditions of fever.

Pulse during 'Vaatic Jvara' :

The pulse moves fast with curve. The pulse is found to be weak light camparatively cold below the index finger.

वक्रा च चपला शीतस्पर्शा वात ज्वरे भवेत् । (नाड़ी परीक्षा)

Pulse beat during Pitta Jvara :

Fever is mainly dominated by Pitta. During 'Pitta-Jvara there is rise in fever and the symptoms of 'Pitta' in these can be easily noticed.

- **द्रुता च सरला दीर्घा नाडी पित्त ज्वरे भवेत् ।** (नाड़ी विज्ञान)
- **मृणाल सरला दीर्घा नाड़ी पित्त ज्वरे वहेत् ।** (नाड़ी परीक्षा)

The pulse moves very fast (Druta, Sheeghra) and in straight direction (Sarala). We get an impulse below all the three fingers but it is more obivous below the middle finger. Due to the hotness of Pitta it seems to be filled and expanded.

Pulse beat during 'Kapha Jvara' :

During this, the pulse moves slowly and regularly. With a serious and careful touch one may find it cold and viscous (Sheeta, Pichchhila).

मन्दा च सुस्थिरा शीता पिच्छिला श्लैष्मिके भवेत्।। (नाड़ी परीक्षा)

During 'Kapha Jvara' there is an increase in pulse rate but it is comparatively slower than in 'hyperpyrexia' Pulse is cold, viscous to touch. Here, fever affects Rasa Dhatu first, which has a similar constitution as Kapha and so with this combination, pulse is cold and viscous.

Pulse beat during 'Dvandvaj-Jvara :

The union of any two doshas results in symptoms of both the vitiated doshas simultaneously. It must be remembered that in such condition the pulse varies according to the ratio of vitiated doshas. The characteristics of predominant Dosha would be seen more as compared to the other dosha.

चंचला सरला स्थूला कठिना वातपित्ततः। (अभिनव नाड़ी तंत्र)

The pulse during 'Vaat Shlaishamik Jvara' is found to move comparatively slowly and is voluminous and rough to touch. It is more obvious at the 'index' or sometimes at the 'ring' finger.

ईषच्च दृश्यते तृष्णा मंदा स्यात् श्लेष्मवातजा। (नाडी परीक्षा)

निरन्तरं खरं रुक्षं मन्दश्लेष्मातिवातजा। (अभिनव नाड़ी तंत्र)

During 'Pitta Shlaishmik Jvara' the pulse is found to be thready, comparatively cold to touch and moves at a constant pace.

सूक्ष्मा शीता स्थिरा नाड़ी पित्तश्लेष्म समुद्भवा। (अभिनव नाड़ी तंत्र)

Pulse beat during 'Sannipaat Jvara' :

During 'Sannipaat Jvara' the pulse is found to possess symptoms of all the three doshas of 'Vaat Pitta & Kapha simultaneously.

सर्व दोष ज्वरे नाड़ी सर्व सम्पूर्ण लक्षणा। (अभिनव नाड़ी तंत्र)

Normally in a prolonged fever the pulse does not remain constant from the beginning to the end but changes according to the condition of the fever. In practice, it is more obvious at all the three fingers but as the fever grows chronic, the pulse rate starts decreasing. A weak pulse is the main symptom of 'Sannipaat Jvara'.

Pulse Beat during 'Vishamajvara' :

Acharyas have defined 'Vishama Jvara' as 'Visham Vishamarambha Kriya Kaloanushanghvaan'. The pulse is found to be irregular i. e. the pulse moves slowly or sometimes fast. It changes the region of identification and even its nature.

पुरा मन्दा च.शनकैश्चण्डतां याति नाडिका।
ज्वरं शैत्यं वेपथोर्वा सम्बन्धं व्रजति द्रुतम्।।

इयमैकाहिकादीनां व्याधीनां जननी मता।
भूतग्रहे सिराऽलक्ष्या भाविन्यैकाहिके ज्वरे।।

(नाड़ी परीक्षा)

If the pulse vibrates slowly, suddenly moves fast then it indicates a fast approaching malarial fever. This pulse indicates intermittent fever but does not indicate viral fever.

In context of the onset of fever the doshas first reach the stomach.

मिथ्याहाराविहाराभ्यां दोषा ह्यामाशयाश्रया।

बहिर्निरस्य कोष्ठाग्निं ज्वरदाः स्युः रसानुगाः।।

(माधव निदान)

In this way, we get a low pulse rate due to the doshas sheltered in the stomach but as soon as they take out the 'Koshthagni' the pulse moves fast especially in 'Vishama-jvara'. Normally when we touch the pulse before the onset of fever, it is found to be hot, and cold at times. This view is also held by Acharya Harita.

उष्णा नाड़ी पुनः शीतं व्याचष्टे च ज्वरागमम्।

The two conditions i. e. going from slow to fast and becoming hot from cold and vice-versa are found in 'Vishama-Jvara' and in Sannipatik Jvara.

Pulse beat during Bhootaabhishang :

Bhootaabhishang may be one of the causes of 'Vishama jvara'.

केचिद् भूताभिषङ्गोत्थं ब्रुवते विषमज्वरम्। (सुश्रुत उत्तर तंत्र)

In fever with this etiology the changes in the pulse during pre-clinical condition are not noticed. In fact, the pulse beats are irregular and erratic, says Acharya Harita.

कृमिभूतविषाक्रान्तदेहानां नाडिकाश्रये।

प्रतिक्षणं विभिन्ना स्याद् गतिश्चित्रा न संशयः।। (नाड़ी विज्ञान)

This pulse indicates incurability but apart from any fatal disease, if we get manifestations as mentioned, then it must be 'Bhootaabhishang'.

तथा भूताभिषंगे च त्रिदोषवदुपस्थिता।

यद्यकस्मात्तदा नाड़ी न तथा मृत्युकारणम्।। (नाड़ी परीक्षा)

According to Acharya Kanad the pulse moves very fast just as rivers in rainy season progress towards the sea.

भूतज्वरे सेक द्रुतातित वेगा धावन्ति नाड्यो हि यथाब्धिगामाः।

(अभिवन नाड़ी तन्त्र)

Different beats in 'Trayodosha Sannipaat' war :

'Naadi Vigyana' by Harita describes thirteen types of 'Sannipaat jvara' with different pulse beats. Normally according to the principality of disorders the symptoms can be seen more clearly in the respective region i.e. in 'Vattadhik Sannipaat predominance is seen below fore finger, in 'Pittadhik Sannipaat' predominance is seen below middle finger and in 'Kaphadhik sannipaat' predominance is seen below the ring finger.

वाताधिका भवत्यग्रे मध्ये वहति पित्तला।

अंते श्लेष्माधिका नाड़ी सन्निपाते त्रिलक्षकम्।।

(नाड़ी तत्त्व.दर्शन)

In this context Harita has described various types of Saanipaat-jvara according to the predominancy of specific doshas, their mode of movement, the name of Sannipaat-jvara, their duration. Yog Ratnakara also has described their symptoms and duration.

1) **Sandhik Sannipaat :** The pulse will be found to be dominated by Vata and Kapha, while Pitta will be low. The fever lasts for seven days.

2) **Tandrik Sannipaat :** *The pulse will be dominated by kapha and* pitta while vata would be low. The fever lasts for 25 days.

3. **Pralaya Sannipaat :** 'Vatta Naadi' will be pronounced, 'Pitta Nadi' will have average speed while Kapha Nadi' will be less predominant and fever lasts for 14 days.

4) **Pitta Vibhram Sannipaat :** The 'Pitta Naadi' will be very predominant. 'Kapha Nadi' will be average while 'Vata Nadi' will be least predominant. Fever lasts for 21 days.

5) **Jivhika Sannipaat :** 'Kapha Nadi' will be very predominant while 'Pitta & Vata Nadi' will be less predominant. Fever lasts for 15 day.

6) **Karnik Sannipaat :** 'Kapha Naadi' is more predominant. 'Pitta Naadi' is moderately predominant while 'Vata Naadi' is least predominant. Fever lasts for 3 months.

7) **Rugdaah Sannipaat :** 'Pitta and Kapha Naadis' will be predominant while the 'Vata Naadi' is comparatviely less predominant. Fever lasts for 20 days.

8) **Antak Sannipaat :** 'Vata Naadi' is more predominant, 'Kapha Naadi' is moderately predominant while 'Pitta Naadi' is least predominant. Fever lasts for 10 days.

9) **Bhugnanetra Sannipaat :**

'Vata Naadi' is predominant while 'Pitta and Kapha Naadi' are found to be moderately predominant and less predominant respectively. Fever lasts for 8 days.

10) **Kanthakubja Sannipaat :** Kapha Naadi' and 'Pitta Naadi' are more predominant but the 'Vata Naadi' is less predominant. Fever lasts for 13 days.

11) **Rakishthivi Sannipaat :** 'Pitta Naadi' is found to be modeately predominant while 'Vata Nadi' is found to be more predominant while 'Kapha Naadi' is least predominant. Fever lasts for 10 days.

12) **Sheetang Sannipaat :** The 'Kapha Naadi' is found to be more predominant while the 'Vata Nadi' is moderalely predominant and 'Pitta Naadi' is least predominant. Fever lasts for 15 days.

13) **Abhinyas Sannipaat :** The 'Vata Naadi', Pitta Naadi', and 'Kapha Naadi' are found to be equally predominant. Fever lasts for 15 days.

श्लेष्म वाताख्ययोर्नाड्योः प्राबल्यं पित्तमन्दता ।
संधिकाख्यः सन्निपातः सप्तवासरसीमकः ।।
श्लेष्मपित्ताख्ययोर्नाड्योः प्राबल्यं पित्तमन्दता ।
तन्द्रिकाख्यसन्निपातः पंचविंशति वासरः ।।
वातनाडी वेगयुक्ता पित्त मध्यमतां गतम् ।
कफस्य मन्दता सन्निः प्रलयाख्यश्चतुर्दश ।।
पित्ताधिक्यं मन्दवातः श्लेष्मनाडी तु मध्यमा ।
चित्तविभ्रमसन्निः स्यात् एकविंशति वासरः ।।
कफनाडी वेगयुक्ता पित्तवायोश्च मन्दता ।
जिह्विकाख्यः सन्निपातः दिनषोडशको भवेत् ।।
कफेऽधिकापि पित्ते तु मध्यवाते जड़ा यदि ।
कर्णिकाख्यः सन्निपातः त्रिमासावधिका भवेत् ।।
वातनाडी मन्दगतिः वेगः स्यात् कफपित्तयोः ।
रुग्दाहाख्यः सन्निपातः दिनविशंतिको भवेत् ।।
वातनाडी वेगगतिः कफो मध्यमतां गतः ।
पित्तस्य मन्दता सन्निपातरंतको दशवासरः ।।
श्लेष्मपित्ताख्ययोनाड्योः प्राबल्यं वातमन्दता ।
कंठकुब्जः सन्निपातः त्रयोदश दिनावधिः ।।
पित्तनाड़ी वेगगतिः वातोल्वः कफमन्दता ।
रक्तष्ठीवीसन्निपातः दशवासरको भवेत् ।।
मध्यवेगा वातनाडी पित्तमन्दा कफोल्बणा ।
शीतांगाख्यसन्निपातो दिनपंचदशावधिः ।।
पित्तनाड़ी वेगयुक्ता कफवातौ तथैव च ।
अभिन्यासः सन्निपातः दिनपंचदशो भवेत् ।।

(अभिनव नाड़ी तंत्र)

Pulse beat during different states of fever

The text books on pulse examination have described the different beats at different stages of fever. Usually with consideration of one or two symptoms, the pulse beat remains unclear but it does underline the serious thought the Acharyas gave to pulse examination at various stages of fever. The specific pulse movement accompanied with other pulse beats during fever helps in a clear and logical differential diagnosis.

Pulse beat during the presence of Dosha in blood

When doshas are present in the blood, the pulse becomes more predominant in the middle i. e. in the Pitta region, it is full in volume and hot to touch.

मध्यकरे वहेन्नाड़ी यदि संतापिता ध्रुवम्।

तदा नूनं मनुष्याणां रुधिरापूरिता मलाः।। (अभिनव नाड़ी तंत्र)

Fever due to infections belongs to this category because bacteria circulate in the body through blood.

Effect of intake of curd, starch or citrus products during fever:

उष्णत्वं विषमा वेगाः ज्वरिणां दधिभोजनात्।
अम्लाशित्वाद् सुस्थत्वे जायन्ते मन्थरा सिरा।
कांजिकया ज्वराक्रान्ते जायन्ते मन्थरा गतिः।।

(अभिनव नाड़ी तंत्र)

If curd is taken during fever then the pulse becomes irregular and is hot to touch. Intake of citrus fruits or Kantjee during fever results in slow beats of the pulse but it does not possess its natural characteristics.

Effect of intercourse during fever:

Indulgence in sexual intercourse during fever results in a weak pulse which moves slowly. This pulse beat resembles the pulse indicating symptoms of death.

ज्वरे च रमणे नाड़ी क्षीणांगी मंदगामिनी।
ज्वरे कालार्त्तिरूपेण भवन्ति विकला सिरा।। (नाड़ी विज्ञान)

Pulse beat during exercise after fever:

Weakness persists even after fever. In such a condition if one walks a long distance, is in tension, depressed due to loss of wealth or works hard then the pulse is found to be moving with different variations.

व्यायामे भ्रमणे चैव चिन्तायां धन शोकतः ।

नाना प्रकार गमनं सिरा गच्छति विज्वरे ।। (नाड़ी विज्ञान)

Pulse beat after fever:

After fever the pulse is weak and slow. It is found to be 'Prasanna and laghu' and is cold to touch. Apart from the symptoms of pulse after fever, other symptoms are also described independently in Ayurveda e.g. sweating, shivering, feeling of itch in the body, not feeling tired, feeling fresh both physically and mentally, itching in the head, sneezing and feeling hungry.

स्वेदो लघुत्वं शिरसः कन्डुः पाको मुखस्य च ।
क्षवथुश्चान्नलिप्सा च ज्वरमुक्तस्य लक्षणम् ।। (सुश्रुत)

विगतक्लम सन्तापमव्यथं विमलेन्द्रियम् ।
युक्तं प्रकृति सत्वेन विद्यात् पुरुषमज्वरम् ।। (चरक)

Pulse during Mandagni and Ajeerna:

Ayurveda has given special treatment to Agni. Agni is considered as the origin of life. With proper functioning of Agni, a person remains healthy but if there is disorder in the functioning of Agni then the person becomes ill and extinguishing of Agni results in death.

शान्तेऽग्नौम्रियते युक्ते चिरं जीवत्यनामयः ।

रोगी स्यात् विकृतेन मूलमग्निस्तस्मान्निरुच्यते ।।

Ayurveda has considered thirteen types of Agni. They are

1. Five Panchmahabhootaagnis,
2. Seven Dhatwagnis,
3. One Pachakagni.

Of the thirteen Agnis, the 'Pachakagni' is considered to be the main Agni because it nurtures the other twelve 'Agnis'. Here Mandagni stands for diminished or low functioning of Pachak-agni.

During Mandagni the pulse moves very slowly like a swan and is found to be full in volume and hot to touch.

क्षीणधातोश्च मन्दाग्नेर्भवेन्मन्दतरा ध्रुवम् । (नाड़ी परीक्षा)
मन्दाग्नौ.शीततां याति नाड़ी हंसगतिर्यथा । (अभिनव नाड़ी तंत्र)

Many diseases arise due to Mandagni 'Rogaha sarveapi mandeagnau'. The main among these is Ajeerna (indigestion).

Pulse Beat during Ajeerna (indigestion):

Ajeerna means incomplete disgestion of food.

It is not only a disease in itself but also the cause of many other diseases. Ayurveda has classified Ajeerna (indigestion) as Aamajeerna, Vidagdhajeerna, Vishtabdhajeerna, Rasaseshjeerna, Dinpaakee-ajeerna, Malaajeerna etc. During indigestion the pulse below all the three fingers is found to be hard and full in volume.

अजीर्णेन भवेन्नाड़ी कठिना परितो जड़ा। **(नाड़ी विज्ञान)**

These beats are found in 'Aamajeerna'. If there is chronic indigestion the pulse grows weak and is not full in volume. It moves slowly.

पक्वाजीर्णे पुष्टिहीना मन्दं मन्दं वहेत् शिरा। **(नाड़ी विज्ञान)**

This is very natural, as indigestion persists for a long period the body cannot be nourished. The pulse during 'Vidadghajeerna' caused due to Pitta is found to be comparatively fast, hot, and soft to touch. It is more predominant below the middle finger. The pulse in 'Vishtabdhajeerna' is similar to Aamajeerna but is more forceful and more predominant below the ring finger. The pulse during 'Rasasheshajeerna and Dinpakee-ajeerna' is found to be uncertain i.e. sometimes it is heavy and moves slowly while at times it is light and moves quickly. Usually these Ajeernas are very unstable and can be cured without medicine and the pulse also starts moving normally.

Pulse beat during Malajeerna :

When the Agni is deficient and the digestion is improper the bifurcation of 'Rasa & Mala' is also not proper resulting in deprivation of nutrition. In the Malajeerna the pulse moves normally but it is thin and weak to touch. During indigestion if the bowels are constipated then the pulse is irregular and is hard and thick to touch. It is found to be expanded.

समा सूक्ष्मा ह्यणुस्पन्दा मलाजीर्णे प्रकीर्त्तिता ।
विषमा कठिना स्थूला मलशेषात्प्रकीर्त्तिता ।। (नाड़ी परीक्षा)

When the food is not digested properly, absorption of is also affected so the stools contain undigested food particles, hence nutrients are found in larger quantity in such an excretion. If indigestion persists then the body does not get the necessary nutrients and the body becomes weak - 'Malaayattam Balaam Punsaam''. Hence in 'Malajeerna' the pulse is found to be weak and sends weak impulse but the pace is regular. There is a small increase in the pulse rate as described below:

मेहेऽर्शसि मलाजीर्णे शीघ्रं तु स्पन्दते धरा । (नाड़ी परीक्षा)

During constipation there is inadequate excretion of faeces hence the excretory products remain in the large intestine where constant absorption of fluid (which is present in the faeces) takes place. The harmful fluid which remains in the body acts as toxin. The pulse becomes irregular and is hard and thick to touch. The first state is found in disease like 'Pravahika' (dysentery), 'Brihadaantra-shoth (colitis), amoebiasis, 'Sangrahani' (sprue) etc. The second state is found in diseases like chronic constipation, piles etc.

Pulse during Aruchi (loss of appetite):

Loss of inclination towards food is an indication of 'Aruchi or Arochak'. Defect in digestive system also results in this disease. During this disease the pulse moves slowly and is thin and free from the Doshic effects.

कृशा विशुद्धचलिता गंभीरा अरोचके मन्थरा सिरा स्यात् । (भूधर)

During Aruchi a person has no desire for food hence such a pulse.

Pulse during 'Aanaah' (abdominal distention):

During 'Aanaah' the excretion stops. Due to the accumulation of excretory products and 'Vigun Vayu' in the gastrointestinal tract, the abdomen is distended with air on all the sides. The pulse in this condition is full in volume and hard to touch. It moves forcefully and is more predominant in the 'Vata' region.

आनाहे मूत्रकृच्छे च भवेन्नाडी गरिष्ठता । (नाड़ी विज्ञान)
आनाहे दृढ़वाहिनी विलुलिता शुद्धा कराग्रे गता । (भूधर)

Pulse during 'Udaavart' :

Due to accumulation of Vaat, excreta, urine, the enclosed 'Vayu' takes an upward movement and causes 'Udaavart'. In this disease the pulse sometimes cannot be felt. When the pulse beat is felt then it is bound to possess shiver and high pulse rate. The pulse in this disease indicates a serious condition.

उदावर्ते विलुप्ता स्यान्नाड़ी कम्पन उग्रता । (अभिनव नाड़ी तन्त्र)
नाड़ी कष्टतरा कठोरगमना तस्मादुदावर्तके । (भूधर)

Pulse during 'Amlapitta':

Due to the irregularity in the diet and present faulty life style this disease is commonly seen among the masses. The pulse beat is found to be curved, trembling, and thick to touch. The pulse rate is comparatively slow.

स्यादम्लपित्ते कुटिला विकम्पनी।
स्थूलाकृति पिच्छिल मन्दगामिनी । (भूधर)

In such patients dyspepsia and flatulence are cardinal symptoms. The main vitiation is of pitta which is supported by 'Vata', but indigestion also exists, so the symptoms like 'Aam' or Kapha are also seen, hence different changes can be seen in the pulse beat. With the increase of 'Pitta' the pulse beat does not increase but it is hot to touch and pulse leaps while moving and is more predominant in the pitta region. Sometimes due to the effect of 'Vata the pulse moves with a curve and it is predominant in the 'Vata' region along with the symptoms of 'Pitta'.

Pulse beat during 'Trishna' (thirst) :

In this disease, even with frequent water intake the thirst does not subside. Certainly it is a pitta dominated disease. In this disease the pulse is found to be dry and trembling. It is hot to touch as found in fever.

तृष्णासु शुष्का ज्वर विव्हलांगी । (भूधर)

With the deficiency of fluids and increase of 'Pitta' these symptoms are likely to occur.

Pulse during disorder due to impure blood:

During this the impulse of the pulse can be felt right from the wrist to half of the forearm or the pulse below the four fingers is found to be forceful (Deergha) and the rate is high.

मध्ये क्रे वहेन्नाडी यदि दीर्घा पुनर्द्रुता ।
तदा नूनं मनुष्यस्य रूधिरापूरिता मलाः ।। (नाड़ी परीक्षा)

Under the effect of blood disorders the pulse is found to be hard and is hot to touch.

अर्केन्दु कठिना सोष्णा स रोगी शोणिताश्रितः । (नाड़ी परीक्षा)

As blood belongs to the pitta category so the hotness experienced is natural but when the fingers are pressed with a little pressure, we can experience the hardness. 'Arkendukathina' word has been defined by Acharyas in different ways. The term using flower of 'Aak' instead of 'Arkendu' is more appropriate. A flower of 'Aak' is surrounded by petal on all sides and is hard in the middle. Similarly during blood disorders, the pulse is soft when touched lightly but when it is pressed one can feel the hardness.

Pulse in Sheetpitta, Udard (urticaria) and other allergic conditions:

As in disorders of blood even in 'Sheet pitta, and Udard' rashes are found on the body. The union of two opposing doshas like Kapha & Pitta' give rise to this disease. The pulse is regular, heavy and viscous (pichchhil). The pulse beat is fast, rapid and enlarged. It is more predominant in the Kapha region.

शीतपित्ते तथोदर्दे समानागुरुपिच्छिला ।
मूला वहति वेगेन क्रूरा चंचलगामिनी ।। (नाड़ी दर्पण)

Pulse in leprosy:

In leprosy the pulse is found to be hard and moving with very slow speed with constant pace but with a missing tendency.

कुष्ठे तु कठिना नाड़ी स्थिरा स्यादप्रवृत्तिका । (नाड़ी परीक्षा)

In 'Abhinav Naadi Tantra' there is a semantic difference in use of 'Sankochi' (contractive) instead of 'Kathina'. (hard). Excessive vitiation of doshas in leprosy results in a heavy pulse moving very slowly. Actually these symptoms are seen in chronic condition. In early stage the pulse as mentioned in 'Blood Disorder', is seen.

Pulse in diarrhoea:

The common symptom of digestive disorder is diarrhoea. The pulse is slow, feeble and cold. It moves like the movement of leech in winter.

अतिसारे तु मन्दा स्यात् हिमकाले जलौकवत् । (नाड़ी परीक्षा)

During the early stages of diarrhoea ('amaatisar' there is an accumulation of excretory products and hence the pulse is found to be thick and very slow in its movement.

आमातिसारे पृथुलाजडा च । (नाड़ी विज्ञान)

As the accumulation of the excretory products increases, the amount of fluids in the body decreases as a result of which the pulse is found to be weak, feeble, cold, but it moves fast. The force decreases radically.

निर्वीर्यरूपा त्वतिसारभेदे । (नाड़ी परीक्षा)

In dysentery the pulses move as in diarrhoea. As it is said that – 'Taasaamatisaar Vadaadishechcha Lingam Kramam Chaam Vipakvataam cha'.

Pulse during 'Visuchika' (cholera) :

During cholera vomiting and diarrhoea take place simultaneously and there is a rapid loss of fluids and excretory products. Due to the decrease in fluid there is obstacle in blood circulation. Hence the pulse is found to be so feeble that one may not even feel the impulse and the pulse may even get displaced.

विसूच्यां दृश्यते चैव निज स्थानं विमुच्यति ।। (भूघर)

The shifting of pulse indicates bad prognosis, but in this disease it only indicates a serious condition.

Pulse during Vaman (vomiting):

Vomiting is a manifectation of disorder in the digestive system. In early conditions there is an accumulation of doshas while after vomiting there is a loss of fluid in body. It is because of this reason, we find an altered impulse i.e. the impulses are first felt in the 'Kapha' region then in the 'Pitta' region and finally in the 'Vata' region. It is hard and cold to touch.

वर्मी विमार्गा परुषा ज्वरान्ता । (भूधर)

In protracted vomiting there is excessive loss of fluid and we get pulse beat as in choleric condition.

Pulse during Grahani Roga:

After diarrhoea if a person takes an undesirable diet or goes for undesirable activities then the prevailing indigestion worsens and ultimately makes the 'Grahani' weaker. 'Grahani Roga' is a structural disorder. Grahani is the seat of Agm. The temperature and energy of the body depends on 'Agni'. Hence in 'Grahani' the pulse becomes weak and moves very slowly. The movement of the pulse during 'Grahani' can be compared to the waves found for a short time in the body of a dead snake.

मृतसर्पसमा नाड़ी ग्रहणी रोगमादिशेत् । (नाड़ी परीक्षा)

The pulse is found to be cold, soft and thin with slow movements.

Pulse beat in Arsha (piles):

Indigestion with constipation results in piles. Hence during piles one finds constipation with indigestion. As a result there is a predominance of 'Vayu' in the body and the pulse is heavy. It sometimes moves in a curve while sometimes it moves in a straight direction. Sometimes the pulse beat is slow.

अर्शोरोगे स्थिरा मन्दा क्वचिद्वक्रा क्वचिदृजुः । (नाड़ी परीक्षा)

The pulse is found to be weak and voluminous. 'Vaatic' character of the pulse is seen predominantly.

Pulse during bleeding piles:

Bleeding piles is a type of piles in which there is bleeding due to the tearing of blood vessels because of the pressure of hard stools. As a result there is excessive flow of warm blood which ultimately causes anaemia. There is a decrease in strength, complexion, enthusiasm and lusture of a person and the senses become dull.

तेऽत्यर्थ दुष्टमुष्णं व गाढ़ विट्कप्रपीड़िताः ।
स्रवन्ति सहसा रक्तं तस्य चातिप्रवृत्तितः ।।

भेकाभः पीड्यते दुःखैःशोणित क्षय संभवैः ।
हीन वर्ण बलोत्साहो हतौजः कलुषेन्द्रियः ।। (वागभट्ट निदान)

In such a condition the pulse is found to be thin, weak and subnormal in volume. The pulse beats are comparatively fast, and is more predominant in the 'Pitta' region and possessers 'Vaatic' character. The impulse may be clear sometimes while at times may not be clear as in anaemic condition.

पाण्डुरोगे चला तीव्रा दृष्टादृष्टविहारिणी । (नाड़ी परीक्षा)

Pulse during Pandu Roga & Kaamlaa (anaemia and jaundice):

During deficiency of blood the patient becomes pale and hence the name 'Pandu Roga'. In this the pulse is fugitive and moves fast and is sometimes clearly palpable, at times it cannot be palpated.

पाण्डौ तु केवलं नाड़ी मुहुराप्यायते स्थिरा । (नाड़ी तन्त्र)
पाण्डुरोगे चला तीव्रा दृष्टादृष्टविहारिणी । (नाड़ी विज्ञान)

It is seen that pulse in 'Mrittikabhakshanajanya Pandu', which is commonly seen in children, is heavy, slow, and is more prominent in the Kapha region.

In jaundice the pulse leaps very fast with excitedness. It is certainly hot to touch. It is very natural in a disease dominated by 'Pitta'.

क्वचिदुष्णा भवेन्नाडी कामला रोगिणो ध्रुवम् । (अभिनव नाड़ी तंत्र)

The pulse is more clear in the 'Pitta' region. In protracted jaundice, the pulse is very fast but feeble.

Pulse during 'Raktapitta' (bleeding disorders):

Raktapitta is mainly a blood disorder in which blood is contaminated by pitta and the pulse is found to be fast and hard. But as a result of excessive bleeding the pulse is slow and soft to touch. In the text we find the word 'Riju' instead of 'Mridu' which means that the pulse moves in a straight direction.

रक्तपित्ते वहेन्नाड़ी मन्दा च कठिना ऋजुः । (नाड़ी विज्ञान)

Due to excessive vitiation of doshas in 'Raktapitta' the pulse is fast, hot, and hard to touch. It is more predominant in the 'Pitta' region but as a result of the ailment, after bleeding, and if there is no further aggravation 'pattic', the pulse is found to be fast and feeble. It is thin and soft to touch. As said in 'Naadi Tatva Darshan'.

रक्तादजीर्णाद् वमनाद् विरेकाद् बीजक्षयाद् रक्तसृतेर्निबन्धनात् ।
सम्मूर्च्छनाद्यै र्जठराग्निमान्द्यात् नाडी वहेत्तन्तुचला च जन्तोः ।।
(नाड़ी तत्व दर्शन)

According to 'Naadi Gyaan Tarangini' during leucorrhoea and Raktapitta the pulse is found to be nodular.

"श्वेते प्रदरे रक्तपित्ते च ग्रंथिवत् ...."

Pulse during 'Vata-Rakta' :

This is also a blood related ailment (gout.) but due to vitiation of 'Vata' the pulse rate is comparativelys low and pulse moves in a curve and may be hard, or sometimes soft to touch.

वातरक्ते च मन्दा स्यात् वक्रता कठिना मृदुः ।
(अभिनव नाड़ी तंत्र)

According to Acharya Kanad, along with these symptoms the pulse moves in a spiral.

नाड़ी स्थिरा निश्चलिताकृशांगी क्रूरा वलयिनी खलु वातरक्ते । (नाड़ी विज्ञान)

In climical experience 'Vaat Rakta' pulse is forceful and full in volume and moves in a curve but with constant pace. Perhaps the words 'Sthira, Kroora' are used to qualify the same.

Pulse during 'Aamvaat' (rheumatic disease):

Now-a-days this disease is found in a large number of patients. The pulse in this case is expanded, heavy and moves with low quivers, in a slow pace. It is full in volume and is slippery to touch.

स्यादामवाते स्फुरिता विकम्पनी गम्भीरता मन्दगता च पिच्छिला । (नाड़ी विज्ञान)

The pulse beats are also stable and pulse moves slowly with a constant pace.

आमवाते स्थिरा नाड़ी भवत्यस्येति निश्चितम् । (अभिनव नाड़ी तन्त्र)

Pulse beat in Prameha (diabetes):

According to Acharya Kanaad the pulse is nodular in touch.

प्रमेह ग्रंथि रूपा सा .... । (नाड़ी विज्ञान)

According to Acharya Ravana the pulse seems to be stiff. It is thin but fills up at times.

प्रमेहे च जडा सूक्ष्मा मृदुराप्यायते सिरा । (नाड़ी परीक्षा)

Actually the pulse is not found to be same in twenty types of 'Prameha' and being a kapha dominated disease the pulse is slow, is cold and soft to touch. Due to polyurea when the patient passess excess urine the pulse is found to be thin and when the patient passes urine in normal quantity the pulse is found with average volume. In lean and thin diabetic patients the pulse is found to be feeble and weak. It is soft to touch. In diabetic patient the pulse moves comparatively fast, is hard and viscous to touch. In chronic condition it becomes obvious in all the three regions.

Pulse beat in 'Mutraghaat' :

In 'Mutraghaat' the pulse moves with varying speed along with quiver i.e. it leaps.

मूत्राघाते मुहुर्भेदे स्फुरणैः सहगच्छति । (नाड़ी विज्ञान)
मूत्राघाते मुहुर्भेदे स्फुरणे संप्लुता भवेत् । (नाडी परीक्षा)

During Mutraghaat the pulse is prominent below all the three fingers especially under the middle finger where its' leaps are clear and is also full in volume.

Pulse in 'Mutrakrichchha' :

मूत्रकृच्छे च भवेन्नाड़ी गरिष्ठता ।

(नाड़ी परीक्षा)

During 'Mutrakrichchha' the pulse is full in volume (Poorna) and moves slowly. But if fever accompanies then the pulse rate increases. 'Mutraghaat, Mutrakrichchha' are two important urinary disorders described in Ayurveda. The basic difference is that in Mutrakricha dysuria is predominantly seen along with retention of urine while in Mutraghaat the retention of urine predominante with disurea as said by 'Madhukoshkaar' (in Madhav-Nidan).

मूत्रकृच्छ्रे कृच्छ्रत्वमतिशयितम्, ईषद्विबन्धः

मूत्राघाते तु विबन्धो बलवान् कृच्छ्रत्वमल्पम् ।

In Mutrakrichchha a person refrains from urinating due to pain or urinates with hindrance, hence the pulse is found to be heavy, 'Mutrakrichchhe cha Bhavennaadi Garishthataa' (Kanad). In Mutraghaat there is suppression in the process of urine formation resulting in uraemia and the pulse leaps while moving. In case of renal obstruction one generally finds hypertension prevalent, as a result there is quivering of pulse.

Pulse beat in 'Pleehodar' (splenomegaly) :

Liver and spleen are vital organs which play important role in blood formation, nutrition and detoxication. During disorders of these organs, especially enlargement, the pulse is found to be irregular, dry and thin to touch.

नाड़ी प्लीहि भवेद् विशीर्णगमना सूक्ष्मा च शुष्काकृतिः।   (भूधर)

Liver and spleen are 'pitta' dominated organs. Hence its disorders are mainly affected by 'pitta'. It is experienced that during hepato-splenomegaly the pulse is more apparent in pitta region and sometimes moves fast while sometimes very slow with excitedness. In prolonged hepatic disorders the pulse becomes dry and thin.

Pulse beat in 'Jalodar' (ascites):

An accumulation of fluid in the peritonial cavity is termed Jalodar. According to modern medicine malnutrition, cardiac problems, hepatic disorders, renal disorder, intestinal tuberculosis are the causes of Jalodar. One finds difference of pulse beat in this condition with symptoms of distended abdomen. 'Shushka Greeva' 'Hastapaad' are also observed. If the pulse moves in a curve, it is expanded and weak to touch, with excitedness, then it indicates Jalodar. If Jalodar is accompained with fever then the pulse is hot to touch. Increase in size of the belly results in increased heart beat and respiration. The pulse rate also increases but still the pulse is found to be weak.

बहुभाववहा नाड़ी स्थूला वक्रगतिर्यथा।
स्फीतोदरं शीर्णग्रीवाकरपादौ क्षीणतान्वितः।
शुष्ककण्ठश्च दन्तोष्ठौ ख्यातः जलोदरी च सः ।।   (अभिनव नाड़ी तन्त्र)

नाड़ी मृणालेन समा रसाप्लुता स्थूलातिमात्र बलहीन विशीर्णगात्रा।

शीता बला वलयिनी कलित प्रवाहा ज्ञेयोदरे सलिल पूरित विव्हलांगी।।

(भूधर)

It is experienced that in Jalodar, due to malnutrition the pulse is prominent in the 'vatta' region, due to disorders in liver and kidney the pulse is predominant in the 'Pitta' region, while due to cardiac disorders (CCF) the pulse becomes apparent in the Kapha region. In Jalodar it is seen that inspite of the pulse being completely full it remains soft. It seems to be filled with the fluid or water. Due to shorter impulse it sems to be moving spherically.

Pulse during Shool Roga (colic)

The pain experienced in the belly reseanables as if a 'Trishool' is being pierced, hence it is called 'Shool Roga'.

शूलासक्तस्य लक्ष्यन्ते तस्माच्छूलमिहोच्यते। (सुश्रुत)

Due to various reasons there are various types of abdominal pain but the 'Vayu' influences all the abdominal pains.

सर्वेष्वेतेषुशूलेषु प्रायेण पवनः प्रभुः। (माधव निदान)

Hence it is obvious that the 'Vayu Naadi' is more predominant. The pulse in 'Shool Roga' due to 'Pitta' disorder is found to move in a curve and is hot to touch (like lava). while in the 'Shool Roga' due to accumulation of 'Kapha' or excretory products the pulse is found to be full in volume and moves in a curve.

वातेन शूलेन मरूत्प्लवेन सदातिवक्रा हि सिरा वहन्ति।
ज्वालामयी पित्त विचेष्टितेन सामेनशूलेन च पुष्टिरूपा।। (नाड़ी विज्ञान)

Pulse beat in Krimi Roga (worm infestations):

Among the disorders of digestive system 'Uderkrimi' (worms in gastrointestinal tract) is common. Due to various worms, various types of disease are seen, hence various types of pulse beats.

कृमि रोगे भवत्येव नानाधर्मवती सिरा। (भूधर)

It is seen that in intestinal worm infestation the pulse moves in a curved path and is feeble. The pulse moves swiftly in children.

Pulse beat in 'Kaas-Shvasa' (cough, bronchitis and asthma):

Cough is a common disorder of respiratory tract. The pulse beat is very slow and regular.

श्लेष्मकासे स्थिरा मन्दा। (नाड़ी परीक्षा)

In fact 'Kaas' is divided into two categories, 'shushka' (dry) and aardra (productive). In 'shushka' the 'Vaayu' is dominant while in 'aardra', 'Kapha' is dominant. In the 'Sushka Kas' the pulse moves in a curve and is very thin to touch while in 'Aardra Kaas' it moves with a slow constant pace.

In the 'Kaphaj Kaas' the 'Kapha' is dominant and hence we get slow and constant pace. In some books there is a difference of opinion, e.g. - 'Kase shook. ıma Sthira Mandaa', in the 'Kaas Roga' the pulse remains 'Sthira, Manda and Shookshma'. In fact cough is mainly dominated by Kapha. Along with these symptoms the 'Naadi Tantra' describes the pulse to be hot and possessing quiver, hence it is unstable, ---

कासे सूक्ष्मा स्थिरा मन्दा पुष्टा च उष्णतान्विता।
राजहंसगतिश्चैव नाडीनामत्र जायते।।
यथा राहुगतश्चन्द्रः कंपितः किल सर्वदा।
तथा कासगता नाड़ी स्थिरा नहि कथंचन।। (अभिनव नाड़ी तंत्र)

In respiratory disorders due to the deficiency in Pran-vayu the internal respiration increases for oxygenation of the cells which results in an increase in heart rate and this increases the pulse rate.

In asthma the pulse moves swiftly.

श्वासे तीव्रगतिर्भवेत्। (नाड़ी परीक्षा)

Along with an increase in pulse rate the respiration also increases. The pulse becomes weak and excited.

Pulse in Rajayakshmaa (tuberculosis):

नाड़ी नागगतिश्चैव रोगराजे प्रकीर्तिता। (नाड़ी परीक्षा)

In 'Rajaykshamaa' the pulse swings like an elephant.

On the advent of this disease the pulse necessarily swings slowly like an elephant but with the increase in 'Dhatukshya' it is dominated by 'Vata', hence becomes slower, weak and very thin.

क्षीणधातोश्च मन्दाग्नेर्भवेन्मन्दतराध्रुवम्। (नाड़ी परीक्षा)

It has also been observed that as chronicity advances in Rajyakshma, the pulse manifestations are erratically fast, weak, hot, thin and low in volume, due to aggravation of all the three doshas with complications of 'Dhatukshay'.

Pulse beat in cardiac Disease :

In Ayurved the heart is believed to be the centre of consciousness. The pulse is largely affected by cardiac disease because the basis of pulse is the heart beat. Due to the contraction and relaxation of the heart, the pulse pulsates.

हृदयं चेतना स्थानं तज्ज्ञातृ सुख दुखयोः।
तत्संकोच विकासाभ्यां जीवितज्ञा प्रकम्पते।।
(नाड़ी ज्ञान तरंगिणी)

According to modern medical science the circulatory problems are largely seen in the pulse. In cardiac disease the pulse moves swiftly sometimes or it moves slowly or the pulse rate is normal. The uniformity in the tardiness is described as the movement of a swan by some Acharyas. The swiftness is seen in those conditions in which the heart beat is also fast and the swift movement possesses force which the acharyas have described as -'Gamane, Vidrutaa, Teevra' etc. The missing of the pulse beat indicates cardiac problem. Rodhvati, Gatirbhangaa, Avarudhya cha Gachchhati'. All the three terms describe irregular beat or intermittent missing of the pulse.

हृद्रोगे तु भवेन्नाडी राजहंसगतिर्यथा।

गमने विद्रुता तीव्रा क्वचिद्रोधवती गतिः।।
तीव्रा कदाचिद् वहति कदाचिन्मन्दगा भवेत्।
मध्ये मध्ये गतिर्भंगा–अवरुध्य च गच्छति।। (अभिनव नाड़ी तंत्र)
हृद्रोगिणः सुकठिना मथिता निरंगा।

नाड़ी द्रुतं वहति सा परिनिम्नमध्या।। (भूधर)

Along with above variations in pulse beat in cardiac problems, the pulse becomes hard, thin and moves in its position. It may not be palpable. Sometimes it moves fast or it can only be felt below the middle finger.

In fact these specific pulse movements and different pulse rates indicate different cardiac problems. During atherosclerosis the pulse is found to be hard, found mostly in persons suffering from hypertension and coronary disease. If the pulse seems to move at one place and it varies in touch, then it indicates aortic disease or valvular disease. If the pulsation is found only in the middle finger then it indicates weakness of cardiac muscles. If the pulse rate and force decrease and the pulse is found to be soft and is filled incompletely then it indicates cardiac failure. On one hand increase in pulse beat, feeble and incomplete soft pulse indicates low blood pressure, while increaase in pulse rate, hard and a strong pulse, full in volume indicates high blood pressure.

Pulse in 'Vaatic disorder' :

In the various 'Vaatic' disorders, specific pulse beats are noticed, which means that the active element 'Vaayu' mentioned in Ayurveda is directly related to the pulse. Some Acharyas hold 'Vaayu' responsible for the pulse movement.

वायुरन्तर्वहिर्याति हृद्संकोच विकासतः ।
तेन नाड्यां वहत्यसृक् तेन तस्यागतिर्भवेत् ।। (नाड़ी ज्ञान तरंगिणी)

It means the specific pulse beat certainly helps in the diagnosis of 'Vaatic' disorder. In this, the pulse moves in a curved way. It is hot to touch and moves fast with different rates.

वायुना नाड़िका ज्ञेया वक्रा सोष्णा बलावहा ।
निर्मला रोग संकरा नानाविधगतिर्भवेत् ।। (नाड़ी विज्ञान)

Pulse beat in 'Pakshaghaat' (paralysis) :

In 'Pakshaghaat', one side of the body becomes paralysed.

पक्षमन्यतरं हन्ति संधि बन्धान् विमोक्षयन् । (माधव निदान)

In this, there exists a difference in the pulse rate between the affected side and the normal side. The paralysed side has a comparatively slow and weak pulse. It is difficult to palpate while on the normal side the pulse moves in a curved way, purely as a 'Vaatic Naadi'.

पक्षाघाते भवेन्नाडी शुद्धा च पवनप्लुता ।

मंदा चैव च दुःस्पर्शा घातितेंऽगे च नाडिका ।।

(अभिवन नाड़ीतंत्र)

Pulse beat in Gridhrasi (sciatica) :

The disease in which the pain starts from the buttock region and spreads out to the back, thigh and legs is called 'Gridhrasi'. The pulse is found to be thick and the pulse rate is low and it moves in a curve.

गृध्रस्यां नाडिका स्थूला मन्दगा वक्रगामिनी ।

किन्तु स्वल्पा च गतिका पीडिते पक्षगा करे।

उभयोः करयोर्नाडी समानगतिका न च।। (अभिनव नाड़ीतंत्र)

According to some Acharyas the pulse movement is not the same in both the hands i.e. a difference in pulse rate is seen in both the hands.

Pulse during 'Aakshepak' (convulsion) :

The disease in which body undergoes convulsions is called 'Aakshepak'. This sympton is found in various other diseases. The pulse in found to be thick and moves swiftly.

आक्षेपके भवेन्नाडी स्थूला सा वेगगामिनी। (अभिनव नाड़ीतंत्र)

When the patient becomes attack free then the pulse is found to be weak and possesses remaining the characters of a normal pulse.

Pulse beat in Apatantrak :

In Apatantrak the pulse moves along a curved path. It moves excitedly but its movement cannot be felt in between i.e. there is a missing of pulse beat.

अपतंत्रके भवेन्नाडी वक्रा व्रजति चंचला।

मध्ये मध्ये त्यजेत् वेगं यावत्स्याद्रोगिणः स्थितिः।

वेगान्ते स्वस्थवन्नाडी दुर्बला वेगवाहिनी।। (नाड़ी तंत्र)

After the end of the 'Vega' the pulse moves normally but weakness persists.

Pulse beat in 'Aptaanak' :

During 'Aptaanak' the pulse moves fast in a curved path. It is found to be thin.

अपताने तु वक्रा स्यात् कृशा सत्वरगामिनी। (अभिनव नाड़ीतंत्र)

Apart from these symptoms other common symptoms of 'Vayu' are also found.

Pulse beat in 'Urustambha' :

During 'Urustambha' the pulse is expanded. It is slippery and cold to touch and moves slowly in curved path.

उरुस्तंभगता विशीर्णगतिका नाड़ी भवेत् पिच्छिला।

वक्रा चंचलगामिनी न च तथा शीता न चामूलतः।।

(अभिनव नाड़ीतंत्र)

'Vaat' is entrapped by 'Kapha', so the above symptoms are obvious.

Pulse beat in 'Dhatukshaya' :

The pulse is found to be comparatively slow during 'Dhatukshaya'. It is weak in force and is Apoorna on pulsation.

क्षीणधातोश्च मन्दाग्ने भविन्मन्दतरा ध्रुवम्। (नाड़ी परीक्षा)

The pulse during Dhatukshaya and indigestion is found to be very slow (Manda). The word 'Manda' not only means the decrease in pulse rate but also a decrease in volume, force. etc. During Dhatukshaya and indigestion the pulse is found to be weak. In my personal experience a weak pulse is also found in liver disorders and in females with habitual abortion.

Pulse in 'Maanas Roga' (psychological disorders) :

Prolonged and excess intake of alcohol results in psychological disorders ('madatyay'). The pulse is found to be thin and hard to touch and seems to be stiff on all sides.

मदात्यये च सूक्ष्मा स्यात्कठिना परितो जडा।। (नाड़ी परीक्षा)

Alcohol is poisonous in nature, which is exactly antagonist to 'Oaj'. Intoxicants are known to militate against 'Oaj'. Prolonged and excessive intake of alcohol results in 'Madaatyaya'.

ये विषस्य गुणाः प्रोक्तास्तेऽपि मद्ये प्रतिष्ठिताः।

तेन मिथ्योपयुक्तेन भवत्युग्रो मदात्ययः।। (माधव निदान)

Hence 'Madaatyaya' possesses symptoms of 'Oajakshya'. Due to poisonous effect of alcohol the pulse is found to be hard.

After immediate intake of alcohol the pulse is found to be fast, hot and thick but when chronic alcoholic patient doesn't take alcohol then the pulse is found to be slow. Acharya 'Bhoodhar' in 'Paanatyaya' has described the beats as found in disorders of suppressed faecal excertion.

पानात्यये गाढपुरीषदोषा (भूधर)

विषमा कठिना स्थूला मलशेषात्प्रकीर्तिता। (नाड़ी परीक्षा)

Pulse in Moorchchha (unconsciousness) :

The central nervous system when affected by the doshas, makes a person unconscious. The pulse moves as swiftly as lightening and also leaps. The pulse is expanded and irregular.

मूर्च्छायां तु सदा नाड्या विद्युद्गतिरिव स्थितिः। (अभिनव नाड़ीतंत्र)

मूर्च्छासु विस्फार गता विशीर्णा। (भूधर)

In fact due to varying reasons of unconsciousness there is a variation in pulse beat. With increase in heart beat there is a corresponding increase in pulse beat. Deep coma results in bradycardia in which the pulse is found to be expanded and irregular.

Pulse during 'Unmaad' (schizophrenia) :

The excess of doshic vitiation results in mental delusion, termed 'Unmaad'. It is a critical mental disorder. In 'Unmaad' the pulse moves very fast and excitedly in a curved path. It is hot to touch. Unmaad is classified into two categories.

1) Ugra-avastha (excited condition)

2) Avasaada - avastha (depressed condition)

The above symptoms are found in 'Ugraavstha'. In Avasaadaa-avastha the pulse moves slow. The pulse is similar in move like 'Maasa Vridhi'.

सोष्णाऽति चंचला नाड़ी वक्रा द्रुतगतिर्भवत्। (भूधर)

उन्मादे मानसोन्मादे पूर्ववत् स्थिर मांसला। (भूधर)

गम्भीरा या भवन्नेनाडी सा भवेन्मांसवाहिनी। (नाड़ी परीक्षा)

Pulse during Apasmaar (epilepsy) :

'Apgatah Smritiryasmin Sa Apasmaarah': In this disorder a patient gets attacks of convulsions but after the attacks the patient does not remember the events during fits.

In 'Apasmaar' the pulse is found to be weak but it moves fast.

अपस्मारवती नाड़ी क्षीणा च द्रुतवाहिनी।

अगम्या गतिशीला वा वेगकाले धरा स्मृता।। (नाड़ी विज्ञान)

Apasmaar is classified in two states :

1) Veg Kaal (active phase)

2) Aveg Kaal (silent phase).

The above symptoms are found in Aveg Kaal or after the fits. During Veg Kaal the pulse moves very fast and sometimes there is missing of beat.

Pulse beat in obstetris :

Ayurveda contains ample reference regarding obstetric disorders. When there is a separate mode for pulse examination of women then it is logical to discuss their ailments separately. Normally the pulse in women is comparatively slow, soft and cold to touch. These have to be taken into consideration during their pulse examination.

Pulse during 'Shveta Pradar' (leucorrhoea) :

This disease is commonly found in women where the pulse remains nodular and is located in one region. It is seen to be more conspicuous in the Kapha region. In chromic leucorrhoea, the pulse becomes 'Apoorna', swift, weak and correlation between the heart beat and the pulse beat is disturbed.

प्रदरे रक्तपित्ते च श्वेते ग्रंथिवदर्च्छति। (नाड़ी ज्ञान तरंगिणी)
प्रदरे दीर्घकाले च नाडी शून्या शुभा द्रुता।
हृत्स्पंदनेऽपि भिन्ना स्याद् दुर्बला पांडुरोगवत्।। (अभिनव नाड़ीतंत्र)

The pulse of women who seem to be physically fit but suffering from this disease, is also found weak. This is a common finding in leucorrhorea.

Pulse in 'Rakta Pradar' (menorrhagia):

During 'Rakta Pradar' the pulse is hot to touch and the pulse moves weakly and slowly. It is more prominent in the 'Pitta' region.

असृग्दरे मंदगतिका दुर्बला साग्नितुल्या। (अभिनव नाड़ी तंत्र)

Pulse in 'Somroga' :

In 'Somroga' the pulse is very weak and moves slowly but after excessive white discharge the pulse becomes very weak and moves swiftly.

सोम रोगे तु क्षीणा स्यात्तथा च मन्दगामिनी।

स्रात्रावे दुर्गंधतेऽधिक्ये निर्बला चपला च सा।। (अभिनव नाड़ीतंत्र)

Pulse in gynaecological disorders :

During gynaecological disorders, the pulse moves slowly with hard and thick touch. Normally it is more predominant in the Kapha region.

योनिव्यापत्सु सर्वासु नाड़ी पृथुलगामिनी।

मृदुवेगा च स्पर्शान्त्ता कठिना सर्वतः स्मृता।। (अभिनव नाड़ी तंत्र)

During infective gynaecological disorders along with feverish symptoms the pulse moves swiftly and is more predominant in the 'Pitta' region. It is thick and hard to touch.

Pulse in Yonikand :

In uterine prolapse the cervix of the uterus descends in the vaginal region, termed, as 'Yonikand Vyadhi'. The pulse moves very fast or sometimes may move very slowly.

कन्दे याते प्रयाता बहुलबहुला मन्दमन्दक्रमेण। (अभिनव नाड़ी तंत्र)

Pulse beat during pregnancy :

During pregnancy the pulse moves heavily showing 'Vaatic symptoms' i.e. pulse moves in a curved way. During early pregnancy (till 3 months) the pulse beat is found more prominant below the Pitta region and after 3 months the pulse is prominant in the Vata region. On the basis of 'Vayu & Pitta Naadi', the period of pregnancy i.e. number of months or days can be ascertained. If suddenly the pulse becomes prominant in the pitta region with other symptoms of 'Pitta Naadi' and the pulse moves slowly, then it indicates foetal death.

गुर्वीं वातवहां नार्डीं गर्भेण सह लक्षयेत्।

पित्तवायोस्तत्र वाच्या लघुना गौरवेण च।।

आमपक्वविभागाश्च दिनमासादिकं बुधैः।

सैव पित्तवहा लघ्वी नष्टगर्भा वदेच्च ताम्।।

(नाड़ी परीक्षा)

Many physicians were able to detect pregnancy, foetal gender, the state of foetus, abortion etc. by examining the pulse. Acharya Vishwanath Dwivedi in preface to his book 'Abhinav Naadi Tantra' mentions about late Vd. Satyanarayan Shastri who was able to determine the serial number of pregnancy; the number of abortions by examining the pulse. This is certainly very astonishing.

This is very clear that on the basis of brief references, available in texts, total knowledge about the pregnancy by mere pulse examination is not possible. One has to depend on practical experience and the grace of a Guru.

During pregnancy 3 months are required for advent of foetal symptoms and after this the maturity of foetus takes place. These conditions are described as 'Aam and Pakva Avastha' in Ayurveda.

During the first three months the pulse moves heavily and slowly in the vata region and then the pulse rate becomes comparatively slow. Clear movement is seen in 'pitta region'.

गर्भे जाते तु क्षीणा स्यान्मन्दा च युग्मस्पंदिका ।
मासे गते चतुर्थेतु स्पष्टस्पन्दा हि नाडिका ।।
अन्यथा स्थिरगम्भीरा आतृतीये तु मासिके ।
ज्ञायते भूरि स्पन्दा च वातिभ्रान्तियुता च सा ।।

(अभिन्व नाड़ीनतंत्र)

It is on this basis that the period of pregnancy can be known. 'Double impulse' is also a characteristic feature of pulse during pregnancy.

Death of foetus is a very serious condition. The pulse becomes very light, swift and is predominant in the 'pitta' region. It is also very thin and soft like skin.

नष्टगर्भे च क्षीणे च रक्ते सा पित्तवाहिनी ।
लघ्वी मंदगतिका स्यात् स्पर्शे त्वङ्‌ मृदुतान्विता ।।

(अभिनव नाड़ीतंत्र)

13

Asaadhyata Soochak Naadi Gati (Pulse indicating incurability)

Ayurvedic Acharyas have described the incurability of diseases in detail. The knowledge of curability and incurability is very essential in medical examination to ascertain and confirm the test and in protecting the reputation of the physician. The pulse indicating the incurability and death have been discussed in various Ayurvedic texts.

Along with various time specifications the `Asaadhyata' indicating pulse has been described in Shastras viz. `Prahar, Jwaalaavadhi, Sadyomaarak, Sardhprahar, Padprahar, Ek-raatri, Aho-raatri, Tridivasavadhi, Saptaaraatri, Paksha and Maas' etc. Behind this lies the divine knowledge and experience of the Rishis. Many physicians were famous for even predicting the time of death by noticing even the very ordinary symptoms. A critical knowledge of pulse examination can certainly help in such pronouncement. Various other physical signs and symptoms which signal death have been described in Ayurveda and termed `Arishta'.

"नियत मरण ख्यापकं लिंगमरिष्टम्" (मधुकोष)

These symptoms indicating certain death have been carefully compiled by the Acharyas. Certain symptoms of `Arishta' do develop before the death of the patient, as there can be no fruit without a flower, no rain without clouds, similarly `Arishta' symptoms do develop before the death of the patient.

पुष्पं यथा पूर्वरूपं फलस्येदं भविष्यतः ।
तथा लिंगमरिष्टाख्यं पूर्वरूपं मरिष्यतः ।। (च. इ. 2/3)

From the above example it is seen that it is very necessary for a physician to have the knowledge of the serious conditions indicated by the pulse.

Due to error of judgement it is quite possible to infer a bad prognosis even if there is no such situation and to take it as normal when the condition of a patient deteriorates resulting in the death.

मिथ्यादृष्टमरिष्टाभं अनरिष्टमजानता ।
अरिष्टं वाऽप्य संबुद्धमेतत् प्रज्ञापराधजम् ।। (च. इ. 2/6)

Ayurveda and various texts on 'Nadi' have described the changes in the pulse which indicate incurability and even death. On critical analysis we find that some changes in pulse indicate definite death but certain changes are very unclear or they do not `clearly' indicate `Arishta' symptoms but only the `Asaadhyataa' or the serious condition of a patient. In this way the symptoms of the pulse are divided into 3 categories--

1. Nishchit Mrityu shoochak. (Pulse indicating certain death).
2. Asaadhyataa soochak (Pulse indicating incurability).
3. Krichhasaadhyataa soochak (pulse indicating a difficult situation).

The change in pulse indicating certain death are of two types.

1. Aniyat Mrityu soochak (Pulse signalling death),
2. Niyat Mrityu soochak (Pulse signalling definite time of death).

I. Nishchit Mrityu Soochak (Pulse indicating definite death):

If the pulse gets displaced from its position then it indicates definite death.

हन्ति च स्थानविच्युता । (नाड़ी परीक्षा)

According to some Acharyas a displaced pulse indicates an immediate death i.e. the patient would die very soon.

स्थान च्युतिश्च नाड़ीनां सद्यो मरणहेतवः । (हारीत)

According to `Naadi Darpana' even though symptoms indicating `Asaadhyataa' are found, but if the pulse is not displaced then `Asaadhyataa' does not exist.

स्वस्थानाच्चयवनं यावत् धमन्यां नोपजायते ।
तदा तच्चिन्ह सत्वेऽपि नासाध्यत्वमिति स्थितिः ।। (नाड़ी दर्पण)

In cholera a displaced pulse does not indicate `Arishta' or bad prognosis.

If there is a quiver in a feeble and thready pulse then it indicates definite death.

कम्पते स्पन्दते तन्तुवत् पुनश्चाङ्गुलिं स्पृशेत् ।
तामसाध्यां विजानीयान्नाडीं दूरेण वर्जयेत् ।। (नाड़ी परीक्षा)

If the body temperature is high while the pulse is comparatively cold or if the body is cold while the pulse is hot to touch and the pulse moves with varying speed, it indicates death.

महातापेऽपि शीतत्वं शीतत्वे तापिता सिरा ।
नाना विधि गतिर्यस्य तस्य मृत्युर्नसंशयः ।। (नाडी विज्ञान)

Apart from this the nature of pulse indicating death with time of death in different ailments have also been described. As in `Sannipaat Jvara', if the pulse is cold or hot and is very thin and moves fast then it indicates certain death.

The pulse which is very cold and viscous to touch signals the death of a patient suffering from `Sannipaat Jvara'. In this way the pulse which moves fast and is very cold certainly accounts for the death of the patient.

सन्निपातधरा नाडी शीतोष्णाभ्यां गतौ स्फुटा ।
अतितन्वी सुवेगा च सन्निपाते प्रशाम्यति ।
शीतला स्निग्धवेगा च रोगिणस्तस्य मारिका ।।
स्थित्वा स्थित्वा चलन्ती या सा स्मृता प्राणनाशिनी ।
अतितीक्ष्णा च शीता च जीवितं हन्त्यसंशयम् ।।
(नाड़ी परीक्षा)

The treatment of `Sannipaat Jvara' has been described as a `battle' with death - `Mrityunaa Sah Yuddhavyam Sannipaatam Chikitsite'. It is also seen that the patient suffering from `Sannipaat Jvara' is haunted with a fear of death. Along with these pulse symptoms, the whole body of the patient is also found to be either cold or hot. In the above shlokas two contrast pulses (hot or cold) have been considered as indicating incurability which also indicate the serious condition of the doshas simultaneously.

2) Asaadhyataa Soochak 'Naadi' (Pulse indicating incurability):

If the pulse is very thin and moves fast with varying speeds, moves heavily, is moist to touch, becomes nonpulsating time and again, it indicates incurability.

अतिसूक्ष्मा पृथक् शीघ्रा सवेगाभारिताऽर्दिका ।
भूत्वा – भूत्वा म्रियेतैव तदा विद्यादसाध्यताम् ।। (नाड़ी परीक्षा)

The pulse which is highly raised and sometimes swift and at times slow, becomes inert like muscular pulse, is thin in touch and moves in a curved way then it also indicates incurability.

याऽत्युच्चकाऽस्थिरा या च या चेयं मांसवाहिनी ।
याऽति सूक्ष्मा च वक्रा च तामसाध्यां विनिर्दिशेत् ।। (नाड़ी विज्ञान)

In fact even if the factors (diseases) responsible for such symptoms are not seen in the body still the presence of such a pulse indicates incurability. Apart from this there are many more changes in pulse which indicate/incurability. For example: if the pulse moves very fast while sometimes it moves slowly, it may stop and then again starts moving i.e. the rhythm of the beats is broken, the pulse may be thin or thick at times, then the disease must be considered as incurable.

On examining, the visualised pulsation with rapid movement on the wrist also indicates incurability. On touching if the pulse is found to be slippery and moving swiftly then it indicates incurability.

क्वचिन्मन्दां क्वचित्तीव्रां त्रुटितां वहते क्वचित् ।
क्वचित्सूक्ष्मां क्वचित्स्थूलां नाड्यसाध्यगदे गतिम् ।
त्वगूर्ध्वं दृश्यते नाडी प्रवहेदतिचञ्चला ।। (नाड़ी परीक्षा)

Earlier it was said that by examining the pulse one can determine the prognosis of the disease. The knowledge of the pulse indicating incurability is very essential for the protection of a physician's reputation. Various symptoms of such a pulse have been discussed in various books. Many physicians became famous because they were able to tell the time of death of the patient by examining the pulse. The disturbance in nature of the heart beat, and the blood circulation influences the pulse which indicates irregularity. The increase or decrease in swiftness and its persistence for a long time indicate incurability. Average swiftness or tardiness and their momentary persistence can be seen in diseasse which have a cure.

Normally the movement of the pulse is not visual but in certain diseases like blood volume disorder, diseases of liver and kidney or high fever i.e. when the volume of the pulse increases abnormally then the pulse beat can be visualised. The pulsation can be felt clearly not only on the wrist but also at the neck. If the pulse is swift and slippery then it indicates a critical condition of the patient. n such a condition there is an excess and large secretion of weat which results in a slippery pulse.

3) Krichchhasaadhyataa Soochak (Pulse in difficult to treat conditions):

Acharyas have described symptoms that indicate Krichch-asaadhyataa'. If we get incurable symptoms but the other physical signs of `Gataayu' are not seen or the favourability of doshas, season and surrounding also indicate `Krichchhasaadhyataa', e.g. the pulse is very thin and cold to touch it moves fast, then it indicates `Gataayu'.

अतिसूक्ष्माऽतिवेगा च शीतला च भवेद् यदि ।
तदा वैद्यो विजानीयाद् रोगिणं च गतायुषम् ।। (योग रत्नाकर)

But if other symptoms of `Gataayu' are not seen in the patient then it should be accepted as `Krichchhasaadhyataa'. This is because these symptoms are also seen in various other diseases.

According to various texts, if the pulse gets displaced, is very slow, either very cold or very hot to touch, changes its speed, weak, not filled completely and one feels the impulse after applying pressure then it should be treated as `Krichchhasaadhyataa Soochak Naadi'.

(*i*) Aniyat Mrityu Soochak Naadi Gati (Pulse indicating death) :

In the `Saadhyataa-Asaadhyataa' chapter various types of pulse beats are mentioned which indicate death but not the time of death. Such symptoms of pulse are called as uncertain-time-indicaters of death (Aniyat Mrityu Soochak). For example: if the pulse is cold and moves with stoppages then it indicates sure death but one cannot predict when exactly the patient would die.

स्थित्वा स्थित्वा वहति या सा नाडी मृत्युदायिनी ।
अतिशीता च या नाडी रोगिणः प्राणहारिणी ।। (नाडी परीक्षा)

If the pulse is `Deergha', thin and possesses symptoms of Vata and the movements are irregular i.e. sometimes fast while sometimes slow, sometimes strong while sometimes weak, and possesses quiver and has `contrast' signs one opposing the other or the features cannot be related then it indicates an uncertain death i.e. it does not indicate the time of death.

दीर्घा कृशा वातगतिर्विषमा वेपते धरा ।
जीवघ्नी वाऽसमैश्चिन्हैः................ ।। (नाड़ी परीक्षा)

The word `contrast' sign or symptoms has been used as an example to show weak pulse in a strong person or a strong pulse in a weak person, indicates death.

सबले दुर्बला नाडी सा नाडी प्राणघातिनी ।
दुर्बले सबला नाडी सा नाडी प्राणघातिनी ।। (अभिनव नाड़ीतंत्र)

If the mouth of the patient remains open and the physician can feel the pulse on the leg but not on the wrist, it indicates death.

दृश्यते चरणे नाडी करे नैवापि दृश्यते।

मुखं विकसितं यस्य तं दूराद् परिवर्जयेत्।।

(अभिनव नाडीतंत्र)

If the pulse is cold, very thin and it moves very fast, then the pulse indicates an early death i.e. the patient is short lived (Ksheenaayu).

अतिसूक्ष्मातिवेगा च शीतला च भवेद्यदि।
तदा वैद्योविजानीयात् स रोगी त्वायुषः क्षयी।।

(अभिनव नाडीतंत्र)

While considering the symptoms of death, only pulse beat should not be considered but the other physical changes must also be noted. For example, if the net work of blood vessels gets distorted i.e. at every examining centre the pulse is found to be unnatural, tardy and very thin, the lusture of the face changed, air does not enter through nostrils, perceptions get distorted, heart becomes in-active, the senses do not work then it must be clearly understood that the patient is dying and the relatives can be informed about the patient's impending death.

नाड्यादिप्रकरः प्रयाति विकृतिं शान्ति परां सूक्ष्मतां
कान्तिर्याति विपर्ययं च यदि वा हित्वा स्वमार्गानिलम्।
अज्ञानेऽपि हि शून्यतामुपगते ज्ञानेन्द्रिये शाम्यति
सूर्याचन्द्रमसौ तथा च पिहिते पञ्चत्वमेति स्फुटम्।। (नाड़ी परीक्षा)

A distortion is noticed in various `Nadimandals' and other active and vibrating organs. Many times we do get the pulsation at the wrist but not in the neck region hence Acharyas advise to sense the pulse at every probable centre where the pulse can be felt. The changes seen on the face such as cynos is, lusturelessness nosey dehydration, oily face, decolouration, etc. also indicate death. If no response is given by the patient's to stimulus, for example, the patient cannot hear a loud call, the eye do not close when a strong light is focussed, does not feel the pain on pricking, and the breathing process stops, indicate a clear death. Acharya Charak has described various symptoms of death in `Indriya Sthaan'. Some shlokas depicting the above are given below:

सततस्पन्दता देशाः शरीरे येऽभिलक्षिताः।
ते स्तम्भानुगताः सर्वे न चलन्ति कथंचन।।
शब्दः स्पर्शो रसो रूपं गन्धश्चेष्टा विचिन्तितम्।
उत्पद्यन्तेऽशुभान्येव प्रतिकर्म प्रवृत्तिषु।। (च. इ. 92)

14

Disease curability inspite of 'Arishta' symptoms

If the pulse indicates certain `Arishta' symptoms then it must be remembered that such symptoms can also be seen in certain diseases which have a cure and hence should not be considered as `Asaadhyataa Soochak'. If other disasterous symptoms are noticed then the pulse must be considered in its totality.

	Pulse signalling death	Disorders (curable)
1.	Pulse moving in different ways with quick changes	Worm infestation, Bhootaabhishang, Vaatic disorder, urinary disorder, Prameha, Toxaemia, Typhoid fever.
2.	Thin like thready pulse	Blood disorder, indigestion, vomiting, dysentery, bleeding, unconciousness, prolonged loss of appetite, hepatitis congenital heart problem, excessive loss of semen, tightly tied upper arm.
3.	Pulse is sometimes hot while sometimes cold.	Malarial fever, plethora, preclinical symptoms of fever, Haemoptysis, obstructive disorder.
4.	Pulse displaced from its position.	cholera.
5.	Weak pulse with slow speed	Anger, lust, fear, depression, epilepsy prolonged xanthopsy, chronic jaundice, habitual abortion and dysmenorrhoea.
6.	Weak pulse	Chronic dysentery, hereditory diabetes, congenital heart disease, anaemia, luecorrhoea, decreased harmonal secretion and malnutrition.
7.	Pulse - very hot to touch	Leprosy, blood disorder, preclinical symptoms of hemoptysis hypertension, renal suppression.
8.	Missing pulse	Excessive excretion, unconciousness, blow on chest, fear, depression, excessive vitiation of dosha, cholera, prolonged pressure on upper arm.
9.	Pulse - sometimes fast while sometimes slow.	Union of doshas, thyroid disorder, Chronic hypertension.
10.	Pulse with low rate and low force.	Indigestion, loss of appetite, malnutrition CCF, depression, cardiac block.

Reference

1) कृमि भूत विषाक्रान्त देहानां नाड़िकाश्चये।
प्रतिक्षणं विभिन्नास्याद् गतिश्चित्रानसंशयः।। (हारीत)
क्रिमिरोगे भवत्येव नानाधर्मवती सिरा।। (कणाद)

2) रक्तादजीर्णाद्वमनाद् विरेकाद् वीर्यक्षयाद्रक्तसृते निबन्धनात्।
सम्मूर्च्छनाद्यैर्जठराग्निमांद्यान्नाड़ी वहेत्तन्तु चला च जन्तोः।। (रावण)

3) उष्णा नाड़ी पुनः शीतं व्याचष्टे च ज्वरागम्। (हारीत)

4) विसूच्यांदृश्यते चैव निजस्थानं विमुच्चति । (भूधर)

5) उद्वेग क्रोध कामेषु भय चिन्तोदये तथा।
भवेत् क्षीणगति र्नाड़ी ज्ञातव्या वैद्यसत्तमैः।। (रावण)

6) अपस्मारवती नाड़ी क्षीणा च द्रुतवाहिनी। (कणाद)

7) सोम रोगे तु क्षीणा स्यात्तथा च मन्दगामिनी। (नाड़ी तंत्र)

8) मध्ये करे वहेन्नाड़ी यदि संतापिता ध्रुवम्।
तदा नूनं मनुष्याणां रूधिरापूरिता मलाः।। (नाड़ी तंत्र)

9) भार प्रहार मूर्च्छा भय शोक विसूचिका भवा नाड़ी।
संमूर्च्छिताऽपि गाढंपुनरपि सा जीवितं भवति।। (रावण)

10) दोष पीड़ा च चिन्तायां प्रहारे त्रसनेन च।
व्यायामे ऽट्टहासे च नैति स्फुरणतां धरा।। (रावण)

11) पक्वा ऽजीर्णे पुष्टिहीना मन्दं मन्दं वहेत् सिरा। (रावण)
तीव्राकदाचिद् वहति कदाचिन्मंदगाभवेत्।।
मध्ये मध्ये गतिर्भंगा अवरुद्धय च गच्छति।।
कदाचिन्मंद गमना कदाचिद् वेग वाहिनी।
द्विदोष कोपतो ज्ञेया ....।। (नाड़ी तंत्र)

12) मन्देऽग्नौ क्षीणधातोश्च नाड़ी मन्दतरा भवेत्। (नाड़ी तंत्र)

15

'Unani' Methodology of Pulse Examination

Apart from other similarities, the 'Unani' method of pulse examination is similar to that in Ayurveda. There are few minor differences. Many internal and external sources have revealed the fact that 'Unani' medical science has originated from Ayurveda. They did consider the 'Panchmahabhoota' and the 'Tridoshas' while writing or translating the texts. Instead of 'Vata, Pitta and Kapha' they have mentioned four doshas as 'Sauda, Safora, Balgam and Khoon'. Acharya Sushrut has acknowledged 'Rakta' as one of the doshas and even accepted it as 'Jeeva'. In 'Unani' Rakta is the fourth dosha. It is most important as it is influenced by the 'Vayu Mahabhoota'. It is smooth and possesses warmth. Apart from 'Panchmahabhoota' (Anaseer) and the four doshas other principles have also been found similar as in Ayurveda e.g. Oj, signs symptoms, Gundharma, cure, diet and Naadi.

Diagnosing the disease by pulse examination is a speciality of Unani medical science. According to them the pulse is directly related to the soul as represented by the term 'Jeevsakshini' in Ayurveda. The soul in the heart is called as 'Hayvani' while in the brain is called as 'Nafsaani'. The 'Naadi' attached to the heart is called as 'Shiriyaan' which transmits impulse along with blood circulation. The 'Naadi' attached to the brain is called as 'Asav' which is responsible for body movements. With this description the system of nerves and blood vessels becomes clear.

According to 'Unani' view the pulse is found in the temporal area, buttock region, near the knee joint and inguinal region but is very clear at the wrist. The place where 'Unani' medical science was practised had a 'Purdah' system hence examination of the pulse at the wrist became an accepted practice. According to some hakims the pulse of both the hands must be examined simultaneously. The criteria of pulse examination are speed, form, touch, length-breadth etc. Where a change in any one of the above, indicates a disorder or disease.

According to 'Unani' view the pulse is influenced by seasons, exercise, bath, alcohol, water and pregnancy. These must be taken into consideration during pulse examination. One speciality found in 'Unani' science is that, instead of keeping three fingers, the pulse can be examined either by one finger or by four fingers. If the pulse moves below the four fingers then it indicates sound health, if pulsation can be felt beyond the four fingers then it indicates heart disorders and if it moves in a region smaller than four fingers then it indicates cold disorders. The term 'Deergha, Ksheena' etc. are mentioned in this context in Ayurveda. The mode of the pulse examination is same as in Ayurveda.

There are two types of pulses according to Unani medical science:

1. Imbsaat (Bahya gati) (external) :

The pulse which touches the fingers outwardly is called as Imbsaat i.e. with outward movements.

2. Inkibaaj (Abhyanter gati) (internal) :

The pulse which moves inward after touching the finger is called 'Inkibaaj'.

There are three types of 'Imbsaat' :

I. Tabeel (length) :

Matdil (Samaan) balanced :

The pulse which is not even slightly smaller or bigger than four finger is called as 'Motdil'. It indicates equilibrium of cold & heat.

Kaseer (Hrasva) short :

The pulse which is shorter than four fingers is called as 'Kaseer'. It indicates symptoms of cold disorder.

Takeel (Deergha) large :

The pulse which is larger than the four fingers is called as 'Takeel'. It indicates disorders due to heat.

II. Areej (Thickning)

Areej (Sthool) thick :

The pulse which seems to be thick right from the index finger to the small finger is called as 'Areej'.

Deyak Vaajika (Krish) thin :

The pulse which seems to be thin right from index finger to the small finger is called as 'Deyak Vaajika'.

Motdil (Samaan) balanced :

The pulse which is neither thick nor thin is called Motdil.

III. Umak (External appearance) :

Mushreek Umak (Bahirgat) external :

The pulse leaps high and touches the fingers is called as Mushreek Umak. It indicates heat.

Munkhafij (Antargat) internal :

The pulse which touches the finger slightly is called as 'Munkhafij' and it indicates cold.

Motdil (Samaan) balanced :

The pulse which is neither raised high nor low but remains balanced is called as Motdil.

The symptoms of pulse according to strength, rate, structure touch, prognosis etc.

I. Strength of the pulse :

Sabal (forceful) :

The pulsation of the pulse remains forceful even when pressure through the fingers is applied, such a pulse is called as 'Sabal'.

Durbal (weak) :

It the pulsation stops by giving a very small pressure then the pulse is said to be weak.

Motdil (Samaan) :

The pulse which is neither strong nor weak is called as Motdil.

II. Naadi gati (pulse rate) :

Sari : The swift transmission of pulse is called as Sari which indicates increase in 'heat'.

Moojjil :

The pulse which moves with an average pulse rate is called Moojjil. It indicates the equilibrium of heat and cold.

Vati : The pulse which moves slowly is called as Vati and indicates increase in cold.

III. Volume :

Hatmalaa (Rudhirpoornaa) full volume :

The pulse which is full in volumes and moves swiftly is called Hatmalaa.

Khaali (Appoma) low volume :

The pulse which is low in volume is called Khaali. It indicates a decrease in blood volume.

Motdil (balanced) :

The pulse which is neither full nor low in volume i.e. it is balanced is called, as Motdil. Blood flow is constant.

IV. Structure :

Naram (Mridu) soft :

The pulse which gets pressed easily is called as Naram.

Sakta (Kathin) hard :

The pulse is hard to touch i.e. it does not get pressed easily.

Motdil (balanced) :

The pulse which is in equilibrium i.e. it is neither soft nor hard, is called Motdil.

V. Touch :

Garam (Ushna) hot :

When the pulse is hot to touch, it indicates heat or fever.

Sarad (Sheeta) cold :

When the pulse is cold to touch it indicates cold.

Motdil (balanced) :

The pulse which is found to be neither hot nor cold is called Motdil.

VI. Saadhya-Asaadhya :

Ushnavaa :

The pulse which moves at least thirty five times regularly is called 'ushnavaa' and indicates good prognosis.

Akhatalaa :

The pulse which moves with missing beats is called as 'Akhatalaa'. It indicates bad prognosis.

Motdil :

The pulse with only one or two missed beats in between, is called Motdil. It indicates good prognosis.

VII. Position

Mutvatir :

The pulse which touches the finger and quickly moves on is called Mutvatir.

Mutfabit :

The pulse which touches the finger for a comparatively longer period of time is called Mutfabit.

Motdil :

The pulse which touches the finger in a similar way is termed Motdil.

As in Ayurveda Unani medical science too has described various beats of the pulse. The nature of beats varies according to the viriation in 'Vaat, Pitta and Kapha'. For example, the movement of pulse like a snake indicates Vaatic disorder, the movement of pulse like a frog shows Pitta disorder and the movement of pulse like a pegeon or swan indicates Kapha disorder. This type of description is also found in Unani texts. The exemplification of various animals and worms shown by the pulse are also seen in Unani texts.

Nature of the pulse beat according to 'Unani' system :-

1. **Gijaali (like a deer) :** Pulse moves like the young one of a deer i.e. it leaps while moving hence called as 'Gijaali'. It is found during heat disorder.

2. **Mauji (like waves) :** Pulse moves like the waves in water i.e. it moves in a zig-zag way hence called as 'Mauji'. It indicates Soada (vatic) disorder.

3. **Minshaari (like saw) :** The pulse moves like a saw cutting wood i.e. it moves in a stream hence it is called Minshaari. It is found during internal and external inflammation.

4. **Doodi (like a worm) :** Pulse moves like a worm i.e. it moves slowly hence called 'Doodi'. It indicates cough disorders and indigestion.

5. **Janboolkaar :** Pulse which moves like the tail of a mouse is called 'Janboolkar'.

6. **Numli (like a peacock) :** The pulse which moves like a peacock is called 'Nuinli.'

7. **Matali :** The pulse whose ends are narrow and is broad in the middle is called as Matali. It is found in physical weakness.

Pulse during Soada (vatic) disorder :

The pulse moves in waves, hence Mauji. The impulse can be felt one after the other like waves in water. It is called as Mauji because of its movements.

Pulse during Saphara (pitta) disorder :

Saphara represents heat, hence it is hot and dry. The pulse leaps and moves fast just like a small running deer. It is called as Gijaalee.

Pulse during Balagam (kapha) disorder :

The pulse during Balagam (kapha) disorder, moves slowly at the same place and seems to be raised. It is called as Doodi.

Pulse during blood disorder :

The pulse during blood disorder is full in volume and hot, smooth to touch. It is called as 'Mumtali'.

Pulse during 'pitta vaat' disorder :

The pulse moves with a quiver and is hot to touch. It is called as Doortisha or Murtaish.

Pulse during 'pitta kapha' disorder :

The pulse moves like the tail of a mouse i.e. broad in the front and narrow at the back. It is called as 'Jabulfaar'.

Pulse during vaata kapha disorder :

Pulse is found to be short and cold to touch.

Pulse during 'pitta rakta' disorder :

The pulse will be large i.e. impulse will be experienced beyond the four fingers. It will be hot and raised.

Pulse during 'kapha-rakta' disorder :

Pulse is full in volume but moves slowly.

Pulse during 'vata-rakta' disorder :

Pulse moves fast. It is hot to touch and sometimes it is thin while sometimes it is thick.

Pulse in Some Common Diseases

Pulse in weakness : In weakness the pulse moves like a thin wire and moves very slowly. If it gets pressed easily i.e. the pulsation stops when a slight pressure is applied by the finger then it indicates weakness of heart. It is called as 'Matali'.

Pulse in constipation : If the bowel evacuation is inadequate then it is called constipation, which increases the pressure of gases. The pulse is very hard. It is called as 'Murttaees'.

Pulse in fever : If the pulse is hot to touch, raised and moves fast then it indicates fever.

Pulse in cough : A pulse which is vibrant, cold to touch, and moves inwardly then it indicates cough or asthama.

Pulse during swelling : If there is a swelling (internal or external) in our body then the pulse moves like a saw. It is also called as 'Minsharee'.

Pulse during heat : The pulse which moves by giving a push to the fingers is called as 'Matarki'. It is found during excessive heat. The pulse which is larger than the four fingers during heat, is called as Tabeel.

Pulse during cold : If the movement is slow, the length is less than four fingers and the pulse leaps are also small then it indicates cold.

Pulse during depression : Whenever there is grief, or a loss or tension prevailing in the mind, the pulse moves weakly and stops while moving. It is called as 'Jalfitrat'.

Pulse during anaemia : The pulse is slow and weak during anaemia and is found to be thin and low in volume.

Pulse during leprosy : In leprosy the pulse moves heavily, it sometimes moves in a curved way, while sometimes in a straight direction. It is hard to touch.

Pulse during tuberculosis : Pulse is weak and moves slightly fast.

Pulse during jaundice : Pulse becomes weak and short.

Pulse during renal disorders : The pulse is thin and moves weakly.

Pulse during excessive bleeding in female : The pulse moves fast but is found to be weak.

Pulse during slight fever : The pulse is very weak and moves with stoppages.

Pulse during sun-stroke : The pulse is thin and moves fast.

Pulse in obesity : With the increase in fats the pulse seems to be covered and moves slowly.

Pulse indicating death : As in Ayurveda, Unani literature too has given a detailed description of pulse indicating death. Some special symptoms are mentioned here. The patient whose pulse moves as fast as light but stops in between does not survive for more than one day. The patient whose pulse moves fast and is thin and cold, dies soon. The pulse of a patient moving with continuous shiver indicates a definite early death.

If patient whose pulse cannot be felt below the first finger, is cold below the second finger and seems to move slowly below the third finger then it indicates that the patient would survive for only three days.

If the pulse of a patient moves only below the third or fourth finger indicates early death.

A pulse which is cold sometimes while hot at other times and it moves with stoppages then it indicates early death.

In this way by letting the family member of the patient know about the disease and by giving proper treatment a physician can guard his reputation.

According to a famous Unani physician if the pulse below the three fingers move with a natural speed then the patient is considered to be healthy while if it moves in an unnatural manner then the patient is considered to be unhealthy and suffers from diseases such as fever or diabetes which spreads all over the body. If something irregular is found below one finger then it must be noted that the patient suffers from a disease which affects a particular organ of the body. For example, if irregularity is below the index finger then the defect lies between the head and the neck region. If irregularity is seen below the middle finger then the defect is between the neck and the waist and if irregularity is sighted below the ring finger then the defect lies between waist and the leg. This view is novel hence quoted.

16

Pulse Examination in Modern Medicine

Modern medical science does not accept such a wide use of pulse examination as in Ayurveda or Unani medical science. According to the modern view the pulse can be examined at the radial, brachial, carotid, femoral, popliteal, posterior and Tibial Dorsalis pedis regions by checking the pulse or the arterial pulsation. Generally radial pulse at the wrist is examined but for the comparative study, the physicians examine the pulse at other regions also.

Mode of Examination:

Ayurveda directs the patient to sit during pulse examination but modern medical science prefers to lie down. The hands should be relaxed. There should be no pressure over the blood vessel hence the patient is allowed to lie down. If the patient can lie down straight then the patient must be directed to do so and the hand should be straight beside his body. The hands should not be bent, contracted or stretched. The hand now should be turned laterally (thumb up and the small finger below). If the fingers are slightly curved then the beats are clear. A prior information about the things taken (which effect the pulse rate) must be obtained i.e. things eaten, distance walked, time since he slept etc. The pulse must be checked with three fingers for complete one minute and not for 15 seconds or half a minute and then multiplyied it by four or two respectively. The temperature of the doctors hand similar to the patients body temperature or atmospheric temperature gives better results. After examining the pulse of one hand the pulse rate of the other hand must also be varified and if necessary the pulse rate at other regions be checked for getting better results.

Things to be examined during pulse examinations:

1. Rate, 2. Rhythm, 3. Volume 4. Condition of blood vessel, 5. Tension, 6. Character, 7. Comparative study of the other beats with the radial pulse.

Modern pulse examination is based on the above seven criteria. The changes in them will indicate the systemic disorders.

I. Rate:

It is based on the number of beats per minute. The fingers should be kept on the pulse and without giving pressure the number of beats must be counted for one minute. It should be noted for complete one minute. The pulse rate of a healthy young boy is 72 per minute. Age affects the pulse rate hence the pulse rates are different at different ages.

	Age	*Pulse rate per minute*
1.	Pregnancy	140
2.	New born	120
3.	1 to 5 years	100
4.	6 to 10 years	90
5.	11 to 20 years	80
6.	21 to 35 years	72
7.	36 to 70 years	70
8.	Above 70	80

This is not a rigid pulse rate. A difference of 5 to 10 beats can be noticed even in absence of any disease or disorder. This can be due to physical, environmental and geographical circumstances.

Apart from age, other factors also influence the pulse rate. For example temperature, exertion, nature of meals, stimulants, intoxicants, cardiac problem, thyroid, psychological and blood disorders etc.

With the increase in body temperature there is an increase in pulse rate. During fever for 1° (an increase) rise temperature there is a rise of 10 beats. This is the most popular practice to measure the body temperature. But in typhoid fever, malarial fever, influenza, cerebral fever etc. the pulse rate does not increase accordingly i.e. even in high temperature the pulse rate does not increase in the same manner.

The pulse rate is also found to increase during exercise or hard work while it decreases during relaxation or sleep. Hot meal increases the pulse rate while cold food stuffs and drinks decrease pulse rate. Stimulants such as coffee, tea, alcohol increase the pulse rate.

Intoxicants such as opium, bhang etc. decrease pulse rate. The pulse rate is found to increase during some cardiac disorders such as paroxysmal atrial tachycardia, sinus tachycardia, atrial fibrillation, atrial flutters etc. In other cardiac diseases such as CCF, heart block the pulse rate however decreases. Pulse rate also decreases during jaundice.

During thyrotoxicosis the pulse rate is fast while during myxoedema the pulse rate is low.

During the presence of poisonous substances the pulse rate is increased and during deficiency of blood also the heart beat increases.

The psychological condition affects the heart beat, hence the pulse rate is also affected. In excited state of mind such as anger, lust, tension, etc. the pulse is found to be fast and during depressed condition such as grief, perplexity, inferiority complex, the pulse rate is low. Increased pulse rate is called tachycardia and decrease bradycardia respectively.

In this way the pulse examination can indicate many aspects of clinical examination hence the examination must be conducted seriously. If there is a variance in the other symptoms with pulse beat then the patient must be laid down calmly and then examined or by changing the diet, again and again.

Rhythm:

Rhythm is examined on the basis of regular and irregular beats, without giving a pressure the beat must be examined for 1 or 2 minutes. It must be seen whether the beats rise suddenly or not or whether there is missing of a pulse in between. If the pulsation of the blood vessel is constant then it is called as regular pulse and if there is a radical increase or decrease in pulse rate then it is called as irregular pulse. Increase, decrease or disappearance of the pulsation is of two types.

1) **Regularly irregular:**

There is increase or decrease in the pulse rate at every two or five minutes or missing of a pulse after 20, 10 or 8 beats at fixed intervals.

2) **Irregularly irregular :**

Increase or decrease in pulse rate or the missing of pulse beat after 4 or 8 beats as in atrial fibrillation. It must be noted that pulse rate increases during inhalation and decreases during exhalation. Arrhythmia is found in cardiac disorder especially because of defect in sino atrial node. If the pulse rate is high then it is difficult to find out the irregularity but if the pulse rate is low then the irregularity can be detected very easily. Hence the patient should be allowed to lie down and be calmed or should be given cardiac sedative drugs. The heart beat can also be known by E.C.G.

Irregularity in heart beat is a serious symptom, hence the rhythm should be checked carefully.

Volume :

With the contraction of heart the blood goes swiftly in the blood vessels which causes pulsation. The pulsation must be examined very carefully by keeping the fingers and the volume of the blood vessel checked. If the blood vessel is filled with blood then the touch would be forceful and risen, such a pulse is called 'full pulse' but if the volume of the blood vessel is not complete then the touch would be light and soft. Such a pulse is called as 'small pulse' or 'thready pulse'. The nature of volume of the blood vessel indicates many diseases. The disease in which there is an increase in heart beat or contracting power of myocardium then the volume is found to increase unnaturally, e.g. fever, hypertension, kidney disorder, toxic disorder, anxiety neurosis, anger etc. The disease in which there is a decrease in blood flow, heart beat or contracting power of myocardium then the volume of the blood vessel also decreases, e.g. weakness, dehydration, anaemia, malnutrition, leucorrhoea, cholera, dysentry, tuberculosis, vomiting etc. Average volume indicates health. A collapsing pulse indicates a critical situation.

Condition of blood vessel :

The examination of the walls of the blood vessel should be done seriously and by applying little pressure over the pulse. Smooth walls of blood vessel indicate a good health. As the age increases the walls of the blood vessels become hard to touch, hence it is said that as a person gets older the pulse becomes harder. Arteriosclerosis (hardening of artery) indicates many diseases.

All the 3 fingers should be pressed, a soft pulse is difficult to feel but a hard pulse seems like a rope. The confirmation of condition of blood vessel is done by moving the pulse over the bone. The hardness of the pulse wall is found during old age, renal disorder, syphilis, hepatitis, hypercholesterolemia, prolonged indigestion etc. Pulse is found to be soft in children, women and obese persons.

Tension :

Some authors have defined 'tension' as 'strength'. The fingers kept on the pulse for examination should be pressed to such an extent that the impulses are stopped. This pressure applied indicates the strength of the pulse. The best way to examine is to stop the impulse with the index finger instead of all the three fingers and feel the pressure by the remaining two fingers at which the impulse stops or the time interval at which it begins again.

During the pulse examination the volume and the tension of a pulse are studied simultaneously. For example full volume and increased tension indicate chronic renal disorder, hypertension, gout etc. Full volume and low tension indicate fever, infection, arterial disorder etc. Low volume and increased tension indicates cardiac problems and low volume and low tension indicate malnutrition, weak heart etc.

Character :

We get special characteristics of pulse beat which indicates certain disease.

1. **Intermittent :**

When there is a missed beat during its movements and pulse stops, and then again moves normally it is called as intermittent. It indicates renal disorders.

2. **Anacrotic pulse :**

The pulse which is slow, has a low amplitude with a prominent notch in between is called anacrotic pulse. It indicates aortic stenosis.

3. **Waterhammer or collapsing pulse :**

The collapsing pulse rises steeply and possesses high amplitude during declining phase. These symptoms are found during aortic regurgitation. This cannot be noticed when the hands of the patient are raisen hastely.

4. **Pulses Bisterions :**

It is double peak pulse during systole. There is an increase in volume of the pulse. It is found during aortic stenosis and incompetence. Its origin is still unknown.

5. **Dicrotic Pulse :**

At every beat two impulses are felt. Such a pulse is found in malarial fever.

In this way several special characteristics of pulse have been described in the modern texts.

Comparison of pulses :

The pulse at the wrist of both the hands can be examined simultaneously. If pulse rates are found to be different then this indicates obstruction in radial artery. Obstruction can either be external or internal.

If the pulse rate at the thigh is less than that at the wrist then it indicates the narrowing of aorta.

The difference in pulse rates of the two carotids indicates pressure on the carotid artery.

If the difference in the pulse rate persists at the main examining points and other symptoms are not seen then it must be considered as a symptom of bad prognosis.

Terminology of Pulse examination in Ayurveda

1. Soshna — Hot to touch
2. Koshna — Warm to touch
3. Sheeta — Cold to touch
4. Vegvati — Speedy
5. Chapalaa — Rapid
6. Druta — Brisk
7. Sheeghragaa — Moves hurriedly
8. Chanchalaa — Moves unstably
9. Teevra — Moves very fast
10. Vyakula — Moves excitedly
11. Manda — Moves slowly
12. Mandgamana — Moves slowly
13. Manthar Gati — Moves slowly
14. Mandataraa — Moves very slowly
15. Sthira — Moves with a constant pace
16. Shithila — Low in volume and low rate
17. Vishama — Moves irregularly
18. Sarala — Moves in a straight direction
19. Riju — Moves in a straight direction
20. Anriju — Moves in a curved way
21. Vakra — "
22. Plava/Plavayanti — Moves with leaps
23. Deergha — Large
24. Sookshma — Small or narrow or thin
25. Ksheena — Thin and weak
26. Prithula — Full in volume and thick
27. Jadaa — Full in volume and moves slowly
28. Kathinaa — Hard to touch
29. Mridu — Soft to touch
30. Stimita — Cold to touch and moves slowly

31. Pichchhila — Viscous and moves slowly
32. Snigdha — Smooth to touch
33. Vishadaa — Voluminous
34. Tantu Sannibha — Thready
35. Tantulaa — Thin like thread
36. Trutitaa — Intermittent
37. Kutilaa — Moving in curved way
38. Nishchalaa — Moves very slowly and weakly
39. Prakampnaa — Moves with quiver
40. Balvati — Forceful

Scientific terms in Pulse examination

1. Frequent — Fast
2. Quick — Moving fast
3. Infrequent — Moving slowly
4. Slow — Low pulse rate
5. Regular — Moving with normal pace
6. Irregular — Moving with an uncertain pace
7. Intermittent — Moving with stoppages
8. Soft — Soft to touch
9. Hard — Hard to touch
10. Thready pulse — Thin like a thread
11. Full or Large — Full with blood
12. Small — Narrow due to low volume
13. Thrilling pulse — Moves with a quiver
14. Jerking pulse — Moves with leaps
15. Weak pulse — Not strong
16. Forceful — Strong pulse

Bibliography

1. Charak Samhita
2. Sushrut Samhita
4. Ashtang Sangrah
3. Ashtang Hridaya
5. Madhav Nidaan
6. Sharangdhar Samhita
7. Bhaav Prakash
8. Yog Ratnakar
9. Naadi Vigyan — Haarit
10. Naadi-Pariksha — Ravana
11. Naadi Tatva Darshan — Satyadev Vashishtha
12. Naadi Darshan — Vd. Taarashankar Mishra
13. Abhinav Naadi Tantra — Vd. Vishwanaath Dwivedi
14. Naadi Vigyan — Kanaad
15. Naadi Gyan Taranginee — Raghunath Prasad
16. Naadi Vigyan — Dr. Sarvadev Upadhyay
17. Clinical Methods — Hutchison.
18. Symptoms & Signs — Chambirlain
19. Text Book of Medicine — A.P.I. Publication
20. Nabj — Shiphaulamulka Hakeem Abdul Latif, Aligarh.
21. Kenon of Abisina — Editor, Dr. Mzhari H. Shah